Disorders of Sleep and Wakefulness in Parkinson's Disease

Disorders of Sleep and Wakefulness in Parkinson's Disease

A Case-Based Guide to Diagnosis and Management

Lana Chahine, MD

Assistant Professor
Department of Neurology
University of Pittsburgh
Pittsburgh, Pennsylvania
United States

ELSEVIER

Elsevier
Radarweg 29, PO Box 211, 1000 AE Amsterdam, Netherlands
The Boulevard, Langford Lane, Kidlington, Oxford OX5 1GB, United Kingdom
50 Hampshire Street, 5th Floor, Cambridge, MA 02139, United States

Disorders of Sleep and Wakefulness in Parkinson's Disease

ISBN: 978-0-323-67374-7

Publisher: Cathleen Seather
Acquisition Editor: Stacy Eastman
Editorial Project Manager: Sam Young
Production Project Manager: Kiruthika Govindaraju
Cover Designer: Alan Studholme

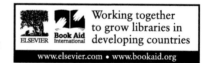

Working together
to grow libraries in
developing countries

www.elsevier.com • www.bookaid.org

Contents

Sleep initiation insomnia

Illustrative Case—1: sleep initiation insomnia

Initial presentation: A 67-year-old woman was recently diagnosed with Parkinson's disease (PD). She reports difficulty falling asleep that began 10 years earlier. She relates that she gets into bed around 9:00 p.m. and reads until 11:00 p.m. at which time she turns the lights off and attempts to initiate sleep. However, she lays there for what seems like hours without being able to fall asleep. She cannot identify anything that contributes to her difficulty falling asleep. Specifically, she denies leg restlessness contributing. She also denies that tremor or other motor symptoms affect her sleep. She reports that while lying in bed trying to sleep, she sometimes gets bored and may turn the television on. On other nights though, to alleviate her boredom, she starts to plan her schedule for the next day, including making a mental list of what she needs to get done. If she had a busy day ahead, and especially when she needed to wake up early, she becomes frustrated and concerned that without enough sleep, she will not be able to complete all her day's tasks. On those nights, she often checks the clock to see what time it is and starts calculating how much time she has left to sleep. She estimates that she can take from 1.5 to 3 hours to fall asleep on any given night, although she does note that during vacations, when she is staying at hotels or friends' houses, she can fall asleep much quicker. Once asleep, she sleeps through the night on most nights. She wakes up between 7 a.m. and 9 a.m. She reports that she wakes up feeling refreshed but does have some afternoon fatigue. In the past year, she has started to nap in the afternoon, sometimes for as long as 2 hours.

Overview of sleep initiation insomnia in Parkinson's disease
Definition

According to the International Classification of Sleep Disorders-3 (ICSD3) (American Academy of Sleep Medicine, 2014), the term insomnia encompasses difficulty initiating and difficulty maintaining sleep. However, in PD, these disorders have different enough etiologies and treatments to necessitate they be considered separately, although they may cooccur (see Chapter 2 for more information of sleep maintenance insomnia in PD).

The time it takes for an individual to fall asleep from the time he or she attempts to initiate sleep is termed sleep onset latency. In general, a sleep onset latency of >30 minutes is considered consistent with insomnia in middle-aged and older adults. Importantly, to make a diagnosis of insomnia, the increased sleep onset latency should not be accounted for by other disorders, which is of particular relevance in PD (see Etiology and differential diagnosis section).

Epidemiology

Most studies that have examined the prevalence of insomnia in PD assess for sleep initiation insomnia using items on multiquestion screening questionnaires, but some studies have also employed interview. In general, most studies have found the point prevalence of sleep initiation insomnia in PD is about 20%—30% (Gjerstad, Wentzel-Larsen, Aarsland, & Larsen, 2007; Tandberg, Larsen, & Karlsen, 1998; Ylikoski, Martikainen, Sieminski, & Partinen, 2015), although some studies have reported higher rates (Shafazand et al., 2017). Indeed, in a study utilizing the Parkinson's Disease Sleep Scale-2 (PDSS2), 45% of participants reported difficulty initiating sleep (Martinez-Martin et al., 2018). Of note in interpreting these numbers, the prevalence of insomnia fluctuates over time in the same patient (Gjerstad et al., 2007). Sleep initiation insomnia diagnosed via interview was not found to be more common in PD compared with healthy older adults and patients with diabetes in one community-based study (Tandberg et al., 1998). It is more common in women with PD as compared with men (Ylikoski et al., 2015). A study examining evolution of sleep initiation insomnia in PD demonstrated a general decline of it over time over the course of PD (Tholfsen, Larsen, Schulz, Tysnes, & Gjerstad, 2017).

Etiology and differential diagnosis

Sleep initiation insomnia may be primary, with no clear identifiable cause, or secondary to one or more identifiable etiologies. Potential contributors to sleep initiation insomnia in PD could include motor symptoms, medication side effects, psychiatric comorbidities, restlessness (including restless legs syndrome (RLS)), pain, and other sensory symptoms. Sleep disorders that may present with (and be misperceived as) sleep initiation insomnia require particular attention, as they require distinct management strategies (Table 1.1; Figs. 1.1—1.3; Table 1.2).

In regard to motor symptoms, rigidity and bradykinesia may make the bedtime routine challenging to complete. Difficulty getting into bed and assuming a comfortable position for sleep can become an issue especially in more advanced PD. High-amplitude tremor may disrupt sleep initiation in PD and also occurs during transitions from wakefulness into light sleep (Fish et al., 1991; Stern, Roffwarg, & Duvoisin, 1968). Importantly, this can also lead to insomnia in the bed partner.

Table 1.1 Contributors to sleep initiation insomnia in Parkinson's disease (PD).

Category	Contributor	Consequence on sleep
Motor	Bradykinesia and rigidity	Impaired bed mobility, generalized discomfort
	Tremor	When high amplitude, tremor can disrupt sleep initiation
Medications	PD medications	Selegiline and amantadine of particular importance to consider. Levodopa, dopamine agonists, and agonist withdrawal are also associated with insomnia
	Medications for comorbidities	Some antidepressants may be activating Wake-promoting medications Medications for attention/other cognitive issues
Neuropsychiatric	Depression	Depression is associated with increased risk of insomnia in PD, and insomnia is associated with increased risk of depression
	Anxiety	Anxiety contributing to sleep initiation in PD requires specific treatment measures
	Psychosis	Especially hypnogogic hallucinations
Pain	Pain	Patients with poor sleep quality report greater prevalence and severity pain symptoms compared with PD patients with good or borderline sleep quality and controls

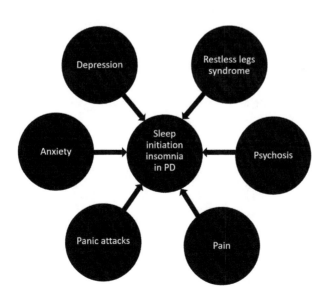

FIGURE 1.1

Nonmotor manifestations of Parkinson's disease (PD) that may contribute to sleep initiation insomnia in PD.

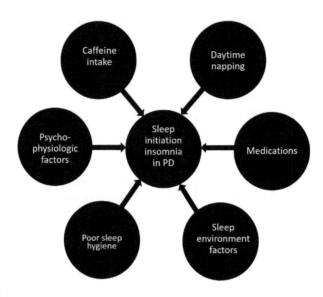

FIGURE 1.2

Behavioral and environmental factors that may contribute to sleep initiation insomnia in Parkinson's disease (PD).

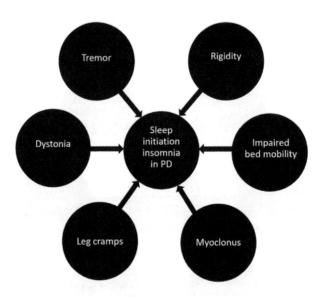

FIGURE 1.3

Motor manifestations of Parkinson's disease (PD) that may contribute to sleep initiation insomnia in PD.

Table 1.2 Differential diagnosis of insomnia in Parkinson's disease (PD).

Disorder	Comment
Delayed sleep phase syndrome	May be misperceived as insomnia when there is delayed sleep initiation at a desired bedtime but not at the "natural" bedtime
Restless legs syndrome	Sensory symptoms disrupt the very ability to attempt to initiate sleep
Paradoxical insomnia	Previously termed sleep-state misperception, this is a mimic of insomnia whereby patients report significant insomnia, but their objective sleep measures are normal (essentially, they perceive themselves as being awake during times of sleep) (American Academy of Sleep Medicine, 2014)
Environmental sleep disorder	Mitigating environmental disrupters to sleep can substantially reduce sleep initiation insomnia

The effect of dopaminergic medications on sleep is complex and may depend on the disease stage (Zhou, Zhang, Wang, & Peng, 2014). Several PD medications have been associated with increased risk of insomnia being reported as an adverse effect in placebo-controlled trials of those agents: selegiline (Lyons et al., 2010), dopamine agonists (Parkinson Study Group, 2007; Stowe et al., 2010), rasagiline (Solis-Garcia del Pozo, Minguez-Minguez, de Groot, & Jordan, 2013) (although some data suggest otherwise (Elmer et al., 2006)), and entacapone (Stowe et al., 2010). Selegiline is of particular note given that it is metabolized to a methamphetamine derivative which can be activating. Indeed, in randomized, placebo-controlled trials of selegiline, insomnia was significantly more likely to occur in the selegiline arm compared with placebo, and it was the most commonly reported adverse effect (Heinonen & Myllyla 1998). A randomized trial of extended-release amantadine demonstrated it to be significantly more likely to cause insomnia compared with placebo as well (Oertel et al., 2017); whether insomnia is more likely with extended release as compared with immediate release amantadine is not well studied. Anecdotal experience suggests that avoiding afternoon doses of selegiline and amantadine both help minimize risk of sleep initiation insomnia. An important etiology of sleep initiation insomnia to consider is the effect of withdrawing dopamine agonists; insomnia can be a symptom of dopamine agonist withdrawal syndrome (Pondal et al., 2013). Should this (or other manifestations of withdrawal) occur, a very slow taper of the agonist may be necessary. Paradoxically, some individuals with sleep initiation insomnia may suffer from daytime hypersomnolence (see Chapter 12) and receive activating (wake-promoting) agents such as modafinil. Such agents can in turn lead to insomnia as well.

Various neuropsychiatric symptoms may contribute to sleep initiation insomnia. In PD, both depression (Reijnders, Ehrt, Weber, Aarsland, & Leentjens, 2008) and anxiety (Pontone et al., 2009; Rana et al., 2018) are common, and both can lead to difficulty falling asleep (see Chapter 3). Female PD patients are particularly susceptible to the effects of depression on sleep initiation (Verbaan, van Rooden, Visser,

Marinus, & van Hilten, 2008). The relationship between neuropsychiatric symptoms and sleep problems in PD are complex. Indeed, not only is depression a risk factor for insomnia in PD, but insomnia is also a risk factor for depression (Suzuki et al., 2009). In addition, medications used for the treatment of psychiatric comorbidities can contribute to insomnia in PD, directly or indirectly by exacerbating other sleep disorders (such as RLS; see Chapter 8). Methamphetamines are sometimes used to treat various symptoms of PD and can increase risk of insomnia as well. Psychosis in PD is associated with increased risk of insomnia (Morgante et al., 2012). Hypnogogic hallucinations, hallucinations that occur during the transition from wake to stage 1 of sleep, may also disrupt sleep initiation in PD (see Chapter 4 on nocturnal psychosis in PD). As for the relationship between pain and insomnia in PD, in a questionnaire-based study, PD patients reporting poor sleep also report greater pain symptoms (Rana et al., 2018), especially radiating pain, painful paresthesias, and symptoms of akathisia (see Chapter 8 for more information on nocturnal restlessness in PD). Among pain domains, nocturnal and musculoskeletal pain are the strongest predictors of nocturnal sleep problems in PD (Martinez-Martin et al., 2018).

A type of insomnia that is not necessarily more common in PD but can certainly occur in PD is termed psychophysiological insomnia (American Academy of Sleep Medicine, 2014). In this type of insomnia, there are learned sleep-preventing associations. Such patients often have excessive worry about sleep. Because of the negative associations with difficulty sleeping that usually develop in the context of lying awake in their own bed at night, patients with psychophysiological insomnia can often fall asleep with no difficulty in settings outside of their usual bed (such as during travel). Identifying this type of insomnia in PD is essential given the treatment implications (see Management section).

Comorbid sleep disorders that present as insomnia in PD certainly warrant consideration. These include restless legs syndrome (RLS) (Yu et al., 2013; see Chapter 7). Unfortunately, in PD, a nonspecific leg restlessness often occurs, which does not quite meet criteria for RLS but nevertheless is very bothersome to the patient and disruptive to sleep (Shimohata & Nishizawa, 2013). A circadian rhythm abnormality masquerading as insomnia should also always be considered in individuals presenting with insomnia, especially delayed sleep phase syndrome. On the other hand, insomnia in PD may in part result from abnormalities in circadian function and the effect of dopaminergic medications on melatonin secretion (Bolitho et al., 2014; see Chapter 9 for more on circadian dysfunction in PD).

Poor sleep hygiene habits specific to PD have not been described, but this factor may certainly contribute to sleep initiation insomnia in PD. Poor sleep hygiene involves habits that are not conducive to good sleep, including but not limited to daytime napping, engaging in activities besides sleep and sex in the bed (such as reading and watching television in bed), and not following a consistent bedtime and wake-up time (American Academy of Sleep Medicine, 2014).

In some patients, no clear motor, psychiatric, or sensory contributors are found. When contributing factors and mimics have been ruled out, the insomnia may be deemed "primary".

Consequences and complications

Data specifically on the consequences of sleep initiation insomnia in PD are limited. In general, insomnia in PD is associated with worse self-reported sleep quality (Shafazand. et al., 2017). While some patients with insomnia have greater daytime sleepiness than those without (Shafazand et al., 2017), at least in a subset of patients with sleep initiation insomnia, daytime sleepiness is not present subjectively (Tholfsen et al., 2017) increased. This may reflect the general hyperarousal associated with insomnia, as reported in the general population. Importantly, insomnia is independently associated with reduced quality of life in PD (Duncan et al., 2014; Shafazand et al., 2017). Studies that have looked independently at sleep initiation insomnia in PD suggest that it has a significant negative impact on quality of life (Avidan et al., 2013).

Management

There are limited data on the management of insomnia in PD and especially when just considering sleep initiation insomnia. The majority of randomized controlled trials testing agents for the treatment of insomnia in PD have had small sample sizes.

A randomized, placebo-controlled trial of eszopiclone in PD (Menza et al., 2010) included 15 patients in the eszopiclone arm and 15 in the placebo arm. Enrollment required either sleep maintenance insomnia or sleep initiation insomnia, defined as three or more nights over a 7-day period with sleep latency of more than 30 minutes. The primary outcome was total sleep time as captured on patient diary. Several questionnaire-based secondary end points were included. Only 12 patients in the eszopiclone arm and 7 in the placebo arm completed the study. A nonsignificant increase in total sleep time was demonstrated. The eszopiclone arm had a 7 minute reduction in sleep latency, but this was not significantly different from placebo. Eszopiclone was generally well tolerated in this trial (Menza et al., 2010).

Two randomized trials have assessed melatonin for insomnia in PD. One did not assess sleep initiation latency specifically (Dowling et al., 2005), but it is further discussed in Chapter 2 (on sleep maintenance insomnia in PD). The other consisted of only 18 randomized patients (Medeiros et al., 2007). Self-reported sleep latency improved, and there were no detrimental effects on motor function, but the small sample size limits conclusions that can be drawn.

Regarding the utility of dopaminergic medications to treat insomnia in PD, there are conflicting studies and again, limited data especially in regard to sleep initiation insomnia. Animal studies indicate that low doses of dopaminergic medications facilitate sleep through action at presynaptic D2 receptors, whereas higher doses inhibit sleep through action at postsynaptic D1 and possibly also D2 receptors (Laloux et al., 2008; Monti, Hawkins, Jantos, D'Angelo, & Fernandez, 1988; Monti, Jantos, & Fernandez, 1989). Human studies have suggested that higher doses of dopaminergic medications are associated with worse self-reported sleep quality (Chahine et al., 2013; Stavitsky & Cronin-Golomb, 2011) as well as with actigraphy (Comella,

Morrissey, & Janko, 2005; Stavitsky & Cronin-Golomb, 2011; Van Hilten et al., 1993). However, in patients with more advanced PD, dopaminergic medications may help sleep initiation insomnia (Ray Chaudhuri et al., 2012; Trenkwaldera et al., 2012), likely when motor symptoms are a significant contributor to sleep difficulties. Thus, the appropriateness of dopaminergic medications to treat sleep initiation insomnia in PD must be determined on a case-by-case basis.

A small trial suggested that the tricyclic antidepressant doxepin may help insomnia in PD but only included six patients in the doxepin arm (Rios Romenets et al., 2013).

Due to the small sample sizes and other limitations of the data, in the Movement Disorder Society Evidence−Based Medicine Review update published in 2011 (Seppi et al., 2011), controlled release carbidopa-levodopa, eszopiclone, and melatonin 3−5 mg were considered "investigational" for the treatment of insomnia, but possibly useful and to have an acceptable risk without need for specialized monitoring.

In patients with psychophysiological insomnia, a structured program, cognitive-behavioral therapy for insomnia (CBTi) can be highly effective in reducing sleep initiation insomnia (Brasure et al., 2016; Qaseem et al., 2016; Trauer, Qian, Doyle, Rajaratnam, & Cunnington, 2015). CBTi is often administered by a trained behavioral specialist (psychologists) but may also be offered by physicians and nurses. The design of the intervention is often individualized to the specific patient but may include sleep hygiene education, stimulus control, relaxation training, and sleep restriction (Edinger & Means, 2005; Schutte-Rodin, Broch, Buysse, Dorsey, & Sateia, 2008). Increasing preliminary/pilot data support the utility of cognitive-behavioral therapy for insomnia in PD (Humbert et al., 2017), although high-quality evidence is lacking.

In a 6-week trial, six patients were enrolled in one of the three study arms: cognitive-behavioral therapy with light therapy, doxepin 10 mg (as mentioned above), and placebo (Rios Romenets et al., 2013). At 6 weeks, insomnia severity score and subjective sleep quality significantly improved in the CBTi group compared with placebo. While patients in our case series were not administered validated scales of sleep quality, information obtained from their electronic medical record, as well as the sleep diaries, also showed evidence of subjective improvement in sleep quality (Humbert et al., 2017).

A pilot trial randomized 28 patients to either sleep hygiene instructions or an online self-administered CBTi program (Patel et al, 2017). Six patients dropped out of the intervention arm, but among completers, a significant improvement in self-reported sleep was noted, within subjects. Of note, the placebo group significantly improved as well, highlighting the importance of providing instruction on good sleep hygiene for PD patients with insomnia.

Preliminary data from small pilot trials indicate that exercise may improve sleep in PD (Coe et al., 2018; Silva-Batista et al., 2017). There are not data to inform whether this improves sleep initiation insomnia specifically.

As for the treatment of comorbidities, placebo-controlled studies of nortriptyline, paroxetine, and venlafaxine provide evidence that treating depression in PD improves symptoms of insomnia (Dobkin et al., 2011; Menza et al., 2009; Richard et al., 2012).

Illustrative case in context

In the case presented, the patient is a female with early PD and with chronic insomnia, manifesting mainly with difficulty initiating sleep. The history suggests some mild anxiety may be contributing, but otherwise no clear secondary causes are evident. Specifically, motor symptoms and leg restlessness do not seem to be significant factors in this case. She has suboptimal sleep hygiene habits, including prolonged afternoon naps and watching television in bed. Her history of worrying about sleep, doing a countdown, and no difficulty initiating sleep during travel does suggest she has psychophysiological insomnia. Thus, she would benefit from referral to a specialist qualified to administer CBTi. In some areas, there are qualified community-based providers available. In other instances, a provider may be located via referral to a tertiary care sleep medicine center.

References

American Academy of Sleep Medicine. (2014). *International classification of sleep disorders* (3rd ed.). Darien: IL: American Academy of Sleep Medicine.

Avidan, A., Hays, R. D., Diaz, N., Bordelon, Y., Thompson, A. W., Vassar, S. D., et al. (2013). Associations of sleep disturbance symptoms with health-related quality of life in Parkinson's disease. *The Journal of Neuropsychiatry and Clinical Neurosciences, 25*(4), 319−326.

Bolitho, S. J., Naismith, S. L., Rajaratnam, S. M., Grunstein, R. R., Hodges, J. R., Terpening, Z., et al. (2014). Disturbances in melatonin secretion and circadian sleep-wake regulation in Parkinson disease. *Sleep Medicine, 15*(3), 342−347.

Brasure, M., Fuchs, E., MacDonald, R., Nelson, V. A., Koffel, E., Olson, C. M., et al. (2016). Psychological and behavioral interventions for managing insomnia disorder: An evidence report for a clinical practice guideline by the American College of Physicians. *Annals of Internal Medicine, 165*(2), 113−124.

Chahine, L. M., Daley, J., Horn, S., Duda, J. E., Colcher, A., Hurtig, H., et al. (2013). Association between dopaminergic medications and nocturnal sleep in early-stage Parkinson's disease. *Parkinsonism & Related Disorders, 19*(10), 859−863.

Coe, S., Franssen, M., Collett, J., Boyle, D., Meaney, A., Chantry, R., et al. (2018). Physical activity, fatigue, and sleep in people with Parkinson's disease: A secondary per protocol analysis from an intervention trial. *Parkinson's Disease, 2018*, 1517807.

Comella, C. L., Morrissey, M., & Janko, K. (2005). Nocturnal activity with nighttime pergolide in Parkinson disease: A controlled study using actigraphy. *Neurology, 64*(8), 1450−1451.

Dobkin, R. D., Menza, M., Bienfait, K. L., Gara, M., Marin, H., Mark, M. H., et al. (2011). Depression in Parkinson's disease: Symptom improvement and residual symptoms after acute pharmacologic management. *The American Journal of Geriatric Psychiatry: Official Journal of the American Association for Geriatric Psychiatry, 19*(3), 222–229.

Dowling, G. A., Mastick, J., Colling, E., Carter, J. H., Singer, C. M., & Aminoff, M. J. (2005). Melatonin for sleep disturbances in Parkinson's disease. *Sleep Medicine, 6*(5), 459–466.

Duncan, G. W., Khoo, T. K., Yarnall, A. J., O'Brien, J. T., Coleman, S. Y., Brooks, D. J., et al. (2014). Health-related quality of life in early Parkinson's disease: The impact of nonmotor symptoms. *Movement Disorders: Official Journal of the Movement Disorder Society, 29*(2), 195–202.

Edinger, J. D., & Means, M. K. (2005). Cognitive-behavioral therapy for primary insomnia. *Clinical Psychology Review, 25*(5), 539–558.

Elmer, L., Schwid, S., Eberly, S., Goetz, C., Fahn, S., Kieburtz, K., et al. (2006). Rasagiline-associated motor improvement in PD occurs without worsening of cognitive and behavioral symptoms. *Journal of the Neurological Sciences, 248*(1–2), 78–83.

Fish, D. R., Sawyers, D., Allen, P. J., Blackie, J. D., Lees, A. J., & Marsden, C. D. (1991). The effect of sleep on the dyskinetic movements of Parkinson's disease, Gilles de la Tourette syndrome, Huntington's disease, and torsion dystonia. *Archives of Neurology, 48*(2), 210–214.

Gjerstad, M. D., Wentzel-Larsen, T., Aarsland, D., & Larsen, J. P. (2007). Insomnia in Parkinson's disease: Frequency and progression over time. *Journal of Neurology Neurosurgery and Psychiatry, 78*(5), 476–479.

Heinonen, E. H., & Myllyla, V. (1998). Safety of selegiline (deprenyl) in the treatment of Parkinson's disease. *Drug Safety, 19*(1), 11–22.

Humbert, M., Findley, J., Hernandez-Con, M., & Chahine, L. M. (2017). *NPJ Parkinsons Disease, 3*, 25.

Laloux, C., Derambure, P., Houdayer, E., Jacquesson, J. M., Bordet, R., Destee, A., et al. (2008). Effect of dopaminergic substances on sleep/wakefulness in saline- and MPTP-treated mice. *Journal of Sleep Research, 17*(1), 101–110.

Lyons, K. E., Friedman, J. H., Hermanowicz, N., Isaacson, S. H., Hauser, R. A., Hersh, B. P., et al. (2010). Orally disintegrating selegiline in Parkinson patients with dopamine agonist-related adverse effects. *Clinical Neuropharmacology, 33*(1), 5–10.

Martinez-Martin, P., Rizos, A. M., Wetmore, J. B., Antonini, A., Odin, P., Pal, S., et al. (2018). Relationship of nocturnal sleep dysfunctionand pain subtypes in Parkinson's disease. *Movement Disorders Clinical Practice, 6*(1), 57–64.

Medeiros, C. A., Carvalhedo de Bruin, P. F., Lopes, L. A., Magalhaes, M. C., de Lourdes Seabra, M., & de Bruin, V. M. (2007). Effect of exogenous melatonin on sleep and motor dysfunction in Parkinson's disease. A randomized, double blind, placebo-controlled study. *Journal of Neurology, 254*(4), 459–464.

Menza, M., Dobkin, R. D., Marin, H., Gara, M., Bienfait, K., Dicke, A., et al. (2010). Treatment of insomnia in Parkinson's disease: A controlled trial of eszopiclone and placebo. *Movement Disorders: Official Journal of the Movement Disorder Society, 25*(11), 1708–1714.

Menza, M., Dobkin, R. D., Marin, H., Mark, M. H., Gara, M., Buyske, S., et al. (2009). A controlled trial of antidepressants in patients with Parkinson disease and depression. *Neurology, 72*(10), 886–892.

Monti, J. M., Hawkins, M., Jantos, H., D'Angelo, L., & Fernandez, M. (1988). Biphasic effects of dopamine D-2 receptor agonists on sleep and wakefulness in the rat. *Psychopharmacology, 95*(3), 395−400.

Monti, J. M., Jantos, H., & Fernandez, M. (1989). Effects of the selective dopamine D-2 receptor agonist, quinpirole on sleep and wakefulness in the rat. *European Journal of Pharmacology, 169*(1), 61−66.

Morgante, L., Colosimo, C., Antonini, A., Marconi, R., Meco, G., Pederzoli, M., et al. (2012). Psychosis associated to Parkinson's disease in the early stages: Relevance of cognitive decline and depression. *Journal of Neurology Neurosurgery and Psychiatry, 83*(1), 76−82.

Oertel, W., Eggert, K., Pahwa, R., Tanner, C. M., Hauser, R. A., Trenkwalder, C., et al. (2017). Randomized, placebo-controlled trial of ADS-5102 (amantadine) extended-release capsules for levodopa-induced dyskinesia in Parkinson's disease (EASE LID 3). *Movement Disorders: Official Journal of the Movement Disorder Society, 32*(12), 1701−1709.

Parkinson Study Group. (2007). Pramipexole in levodopa-treated Parkinson disease patients of African, Asian, and Hispanic heritage. *Clinical Neuropharmacology, 30*(2), 72−85.

Patel, S., Ojo, O., Genc, G., Oravivattanakul, S., Huo, Y., Rasameesoraj, T., Wang, L., Bena, J., Drerup, M., Foldvary-Schaefer, N., Ahmed, A., & Fernandez, H. H. (2017). A Computerized Cognitive behavioral therapy Randomized, Controlled, pilot trial for insomnia in Parkinson Disease (ACCORD-PD). *Journal of clinical movement disorders, 21*(4), 16.

Pondal, M., Marras, C., Miyasaki, J., Moro, E., Armstrong, M. J., Strafella, A. P., et al. (2013). Clinical features of dopamine agonist withdrawal syndrome in a movement disorders clinic. *Journal of Neurology Neurosurgery and Psychiatry, 84*(2), 130−135.

Pontone, G. M., Williams, J. R., Anderson, K. E., Chase, G., Goldstein, S. A., Grill, S., et al. (2009). Prevalence of anxiety disorders and anxiety subtypes in patients with Parkinson's disease. *Movement Disorders: Official Journal of the Movement Disorder Society, 24*(9), 1333−1338.

Qaseem, A., Kansagara, D., Forciea, M. A., Cooke, M., Denberg, T. D., & Clinical Guidelines Committee of the American College of Physicians. (2016). Management of chronic insomnia disorder in adults: A clinical practice guideline from the American College of Physicians. *Annals of Internal Medicine, 165*(2), 125−133.

Rana, A. Q., Qureshi, A. R. M., Shamli Oghli, Y., Saqib, Y., Mohammed, B., Sarfraz, Z., et al. (2018). Decreased sleep quality in Parkinson's patients is associated with higher anxiety and depression prevalence and severity, and correlates with pain intensity and quality. *Neurological Research, 40*(8), 696−701.

Ray Chaudhuri, K., Martinez-Martin, P., Rolfe, K. A., Cooper, J., Rockett, C. B., Giorgi, L., et al. (2012). Improvements in nocturnal symptoms with ropinirole prolonged release in patients with advanced Parkinson's disease. *European Journal of Neurology: The Official Journal of the European Federation of Neurological Societies, 19*(1), 105−113.

Reijnders, J. S., Ehrt, U., Weber, W. E., Aarsland, D., & Leentjens, A. F. (2008). A systematic review of prevalence studies of depression in Parkinson's disease. *Movement Disorders: Official Journal of the Movement Disorder Society, 23*(2), 183−189. quiz 313.

Richard, I. H., McDermott, M. P., Kurlan, R., Lyness, J. M., Como, P. G., Pearson, N., et al. (2012). A randomized, double-blind, placebo-controlled trial of antidepressants in Parkinson disease. *Neurology, 78*(16), 1229−1236.

Rios Romenets, S., Creti, L., Fichten, C., Bailes, S., Libman, E., Pelletier, A., et al. (2013). Doxepin and cognitive behavioural therapy for insomnia in patients with Parkinson's disease — a randomized study. *Parkinsonism & Related Disorders, 19*(7), 670−675.

Schutte-Rodin, S., Broch, L., Buysse, D., Dorsey, C., & Sateia, M. (2008). Clinical guideline for the evaluation and management of chronic insomnia in adults. *Journal of Clinical Sleep Medicine: Official Publication of the American Academy of Sleep Medicine, 4*(5), 487−504.

Seppi, K., Weintraub, D., Coelho, M., Perez-Lloret, S., Fox, S. H., Katzenschlager, R., et al. (2011). The movement disorder society evidence-based medicine review update: Treatments for the non-motor symptoms of Parkinson's disease. *Movement Disorders: Official Journal of the Movement Disorder Society, 26*(Suppl. 3), S42−S80.

Shafazand, S., Wallace, D. M., Arheart, K. L., Vargas, S., Luca, C. C., Moore, H., et al. (2017). Insomnia, sleep quality, and quality of life in mild to moderate Parkinson's disease. *Annals of the American Thoracic Society, 14*(3), 412−419.

Shimohata, T., & Nishizawa, M. (2013). Sleep disturbance in patients with Parkinson's disease presenting with leg motor restlessness. *Parkinsonism & Related Disorders, 19*(5), 571−572.

Silva-Batista, C., de Brito, L. C., Corcos, D. M., Roschel, H., de Mello, M. T., Piemonte, M. E. P., et al. (2017). Resistance training improves sleep quality in subjects with moderate Parkinson's disease. *The Journal of Strength & Conditioning Research, 31*(8), 2270−2277.

Solis-Garcia del Pozo, J., Minguez-Minguez, S., de Groot, P. W., & Jordan, J. (2013). Rasagiline meta-analysis: A spotlight on clinical safety and adverse events when treating Parkinson's disease. *Expert Opinion on Drug Safety, 12*(4), 479−486.

Stavitsky, K., & Cronin-Golomb, A. (2011). Sleep quality in Parkinson disease: An examination of clinical variables. *Cognitive and Behavioral Neurology: Official Journal of the Society for Behavioral and Cognitive Neurology, 24*(2), 43−49.

Stern, M., Roffwarg, H., & Duvoisin, R. (1968). The parkinsonian tremor in sleep. *The Journal of Nervous and Mental Disease, 147*(2), 202−210.

Stowe, R., Ives, N., Clarke, C. E., Deane, K., Hilten, van, Wheatley, K., et al. (2010). Evaluation of the efficacy and safety of adjuvant treatment to levodopa therapy in Parkinson s disease patients with motor complications. *The Cochrane Database of Systematic Reviews*, (7). CD007166.

Suzuki, K., Miyamoto, M., Miyamoto, T., Okuma, Y., Hattori, N., Kamei, S., et al. (2009). Correlation between depressive symptoms and nocturnal disturbances in Japanese patients with Parkinson's disease. *Parkinsonism & Related Disorders, 15*(1), 15−19.

Tandberg, E., Larsen, J. P., & Karlsen, K. (1998). A community-based study of sleep disorders in patients with Parkinson's disease. *Movement Disorders: Official Journal of the Movement Disorder Society, 13*(6), 895−899.

Tholfsen, L. K., Larsen, J. P., Schulz, J., Tysnes, O. B., & Gjerstad, M. D. (2017). Changes in insomnia subtypes in early Parkinson disease. *Neurology, 88*(4), 352−358.

Trauer, J. M., Qian, M. Y., Doyle, J. S., Rajaratnam, S. M., & Cunnington, D. (2015). Cognitive behavioral therapy for chronic insomnia: A systematic review and meta-analysis. *Annals of Internal Medicine, 163*(3), 191−204.

Trenkwaldera, C., Kiesb, B., Dioszeghyc, P., Hilld, D., Surmanne, E., Boroojerdie, B., et al. (2012). Rotigotine transdermal system for the management of motor function and sleep disturbances in Parkinson's disease: Results from a 1-year, open-label extension of the RECOVER study. *Basal Ganglia, 2*(2), 79−85.

Van Hilten, J. J., Hoogland, G., van der Velde, E. A., van Dijk, J. G., Kerkhof, G. A., & Roos, R. A. (1993). Quantitative assessment of parkinsonian patients by continuous wrist activity monitoring. *Clinical Neuropharmacology, 16*(1), 36–45.

Verbaan, D., van Rooden, S. M., Visser, M., Marinus, J., & van Hilten, J. J. (2008). Nighttime sleep problems and daytime sleepiness in Parkinson's disease. *Movement Disorders: Official Journal of the Movement Disorder Society, 23*(1), 35–41.

Ylikoski, A., Martikainen, K., Sieminski, M., & Partinen, M. (2015). Parkinson's disease and insomnia. *Neurological Sciences: Official Journal of the Italian Neurological Society and of the Italian Society of Clinical Neurophysiology, 36*(11), 2003–2010.

Yu, S. Y., Sun, L., Liu, Z., Huang, X. Y., Zuo, L. J., Cao, C. J., et al. (2013). Sleep disorders in Parkinson's disease: Clinical features, iron metabolism and related mechanism. *PLoS One, 8*(12), e82924.

Zhou, C. Q., Zhang, J. W., Wang, M., & Peng, G. G. (2014). Meta-analysis of the efficacy and safety of long-acting non-ergot dopamine agonists in Parkinson's disease. *Journal of Clinical Neuroscience: Official Journal of the Neurosurgical Society of Australasia, 21*(7), 1094–1101.

Sleep maintenance insomnia

Illustrative Case—2: sleep maintenance insomnia

A 67-year-old man was diagnosed with Parkinson's disease (PD) 5 years ago. His daytime motor symptoms are reasonably well controlled on levodopa monotherapy; he takes 200 mg four times a day at 7:00 a.m., 11:00 a.m., 3:00 p.m., and 7:00 p.m. He presents for follow-up with his neurologists and reports ongoing issues with problems staying asleep. He says he can initiate sleep without difficulty, usually around 11:00 p.m., but then has repeated awakenings throughout the night each lasting 10—60 minutes. Each time he wakes up, he gets up to urinate. Sometimes, he can fall back asleep without much difficulty, but other times he has difficulty getting comfortable and has some stiffness and tremor, which he feels interfere with his ability to fall back asleep. He will therefore have bouts of sleep throughout the night, with his terminal awakening around 7:00 a.m. Although he spends 8 hours in bed, he estimates only a total of about 5 hours of sleep over the night. He has daytime fatigue and naps intentionally around 1:00 p.m., sometimes for as long as 2 hours.

Overview of sleep maintenance insomnia in Parkinson's disease
Definition

The term insomnia encompasses both difficulty initiating and difficulty maintaining sleep. Insomnia is broadly defined as "a persistent difficulty with sleep initiation, duration, consolidation, or quality that occurs despite adequate opportunity and circumstances for sleep, and results in some form of daytime impairment" (American Academy of Sleep Medicine, 2014). In PD, sleep onset and maintenance insomnia often cooccur and share several considerations in terms of etiology, epidemiology, consequences, and management. However, there are also key differences. Thus, they are important to consider separately (see Chapter 1 for more information of sleep initiation insomnia in PD).

While a few brief nighttime arousals are common and considered normal in older adults, sleep maintenance insomnia is subjectively identified via report of sleep fragmentation, nighttime awakenings, and early-morning awakening that result in

Disorders of Sleep and Wakefulness in Parkinson's Disease. https://doi.org/10.1016/B978-0-323-67374-7.00002-X

daytime impairment. A polysomnographic correlate of sleep maintenance insomnia is the time an individual spends awake after an initial period of sleep or wake time after sleep onset (WASO). Sleep efficiency (SE), or the time spent asleep divided by the total time spent in bed, is a measure that encompasses both sleep onset and sleep maintenance insomnia (at least, the period the patient spends awake in bed), as does total sleep time (TST).

Epidemiology

Subjective report of sleep fragmentation is the most commonly reported sleep complaint in PD (Gomez-Esteban et al., 2006). When compared with the general population, poor nighttime sleep, as assessed via questionnaire, is more common in PD (Verbaan, van Rooden, Visser, Marinus, & van Hilten, 2008).

In questionnaire-based studies examining prevalence of "poor sleep" in PD, which encompasses sleep maintenance insomnia as well as several other sleep-related symptoms, as many as 80% of PD symptoms report poor sleep (Gjerstad, Wentzel-Larsen, Aarsland, & Larsen, 2007; Porter, Macfarlane, & Walker, 2008; Tse et al., 2005). When physician interview is used to ascertain poor sleep, the prevalence is up to 60% (Jongwanasiri, Prayoonwiwat, Pisarnpong, Srivanitchapoom, & Chotinaiwattarakul, 2014; Tse et al., 2005). Greater PD disease severity is present in those with poor sleep compared with those without (Barone et al., 2010; Gjerstad et al., 2007; Politis et al., 2010). Female sex is another risk factor for poor subjective sleep in general, and insomnia specifically, in PD (Gjerstad et al., 2007; Porter et al., 2008; Verbaan et al., 2008), even in early PD (Tholfsen, Larsen, Schulz, Tysnes, & Gjerstad, 2017).

In a study examining the evolution of sleep symptoms in PD as assessed by semistructured interview (Gjerstad et al., 2007), 231 PD patients with a several-years disease duration were assessed at baseline, and reevaluation occurred in 142 four years later and 89 eight years later. The prevalence of insomnia across the cohort remained relatively stable at around 60%. Sleep fragmentation was reported in 23%–44%. Of the 89 assessed at all three study visits, 83% reported insomnia on at least two study visits and 33% reported insomnia at all three study visits. As for the incidence of insomnia, 18 (20%) of the 89 who did not report insomnia at baseline developed it on follow-up. As for the evolution of insomnia in early PD, the prevalence of sleep maintenance insomnia increases within the first 5 years of PD diagnosis, especially among those who were initiated on dopamine agonist therapy (Tholfsen et al., 2017).

Sleep onset and sleep maintenance insomnia cooccur in many PD patients. One study estimated a prevalence of both in 44% of 182 studied patients (Tholfsen et al., 2017; see Chapter 1 for more information of sleep initiation insomnia in PD).

As for polysomnographic measures of sleep maintenance insomnia, PD patients have significantly lower TST and SE compared with controls. Their sleep architecture is also different from controls: PD patients spend more time in stage 1 and less time in REM sleep (Yong, Fook-Chong, Pavanni, Lim, & Tan, 2011). Importantly, the correlation between objective and subjective sleep in PD is not strong, suggesting that there is some subjectivity in the patient's assessment of their nighttime sleep, that is unmeasured by polysomnography, and that influences their perceived sleep quality (Yong et al., 2011).

Regarding objective measures of poor sleep in PD, polysomnography is useful in identifying potential causes of insomnia, such as obstructive sleep apnea (OSA). One study found that PD patients have significantly lower TST, SE, and increased REM sleep latency compared with age-matched healthy controls. They spent more time in stage 1 and less in REM, but without difference in number of arousals (Yong et al., 2011). SE and TST were reduced in those with subjective insomnia, but this was not statistically significant ($P = .07$).

Etiology and differential diagnosis

There are several possible contributors to sleep maintenance in insomnia in PD (Table 2.1; Figs. 2.1 and 2.2).

These include motor symptoms such as rigidity and tremor (Gomez-Esteban et al., 2006; Tholfsen et al., 2017). Difficulty with bed mobility, such as getting into bed but also turning over in bed and other position adjustments, is a common problem in PD (Louter et al., 2013; Stack & Ashburn, 2006). Impaired bed mobility in PD is associated subjectively (Louter et al., 2013; Stack & Ashburn, 2006) and objectively (Louter et al., 2013) with difficulty maintaining sleep. High-amplitude tremor may disrupt sleep onset and continuity in PD as well (Stern, Roffwarg, & Duvoisin, 1968), as may dystonia (Suzuki et al., 2009).

Nonmotor symptoms such as pain also may exacerbate insomnia in PD (Fig. 2.2).

Neuropsychiatric symptoms, including anxiety, depression, and panic attacks, may contribute to sleep maintenance insomnia due to various effects (Verbaan

Table 2.1 Contribution of motor and nonmotor manifestations of Parkinson's disease (PD) to sleep maintenance insomnia.

Category	Etiologic factors contributing to insomnia
Motor symptoms of PD	Wearing off of PD medications leads to emergence of various motor symptoms (tremor, rigidity, trouble with bed mobility) and off dystonia (both nocturnal and early-morning dystonia).
	High-amplitude tremor may disrupt ability of patient to fall back asleep after awakening.
Medications	Several PD medications can lead to insomnia in PD, including amantadine and selegiline. Medications used to treat comorbidities may also contribute to insomnia. For example, some antidepressants and wake-promoting agents may lead to insomnia.
Neuropsychiatric symptoms	Depression, anxiety, and nocturnal panic attacks may all be associated with sleep maintenance insomnia in PD.
Autonomic	Nocturia is a commonly reported symptom in patients with sleep maintenance insomnia.

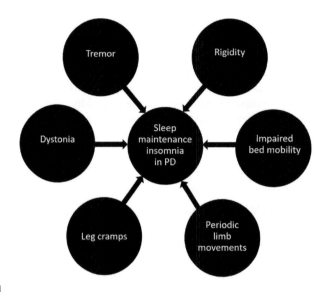

FIGURE 2.1

Motor manifestations that may contribute to sleep maintenance insomnia in Parkinson's disease (PD).

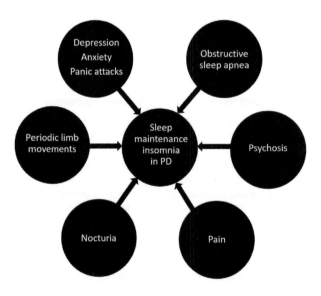

FIGURE 2.2

Nonmotor manifestations of Parkinson's disease (PD) that may contribute to sleep maintenance insomnia in PD.

et al., 2008; see Chapter 3 for more information on the effect of mood and anxiety disorders on sleep in PD). Similarly, nocturnal psychosis may disrupt sleep maintenance in PD. This is discussed further in Chapter 4.

As for medications, some of the medications used to treat PD may cause insomnia as a side effect. These include amantadine and selegiline (Lyons et al., 2010). The effect of dopaminergic medications on sleep in PD is complex. At least in some cases, dopaminergic medications may exacerbate sleep initiation and maintenance (Chahine et al., 2013). However, this may vary according to disease stage (Zhou, Zhang, Wang, & Peng, 2014).

Nocturia, one of the most commonly reported symptoms in PD, is common among individuals reporting poor sleep and especially among those reporting difficulty with sleep maintenance. To what degree the urge to urinate leads to disrupted sleep or is the result of disrupted sleep is not clear and deserves further study. Anecdotally, treatment of nocturia in PD does lead to improved sleep at least in some cases. On the other hand, treatment of insomnia in PD also seems to reduce the frequency of nocturia in some patients, although data on this are limited (see Chapter 10 for more information on nocturia in PD).

Comorbid sleep disorders such as sleep apnea and periodic limb movement disorder may also lead to sleep fragmentation. Therefore, polysomnography is indicated in the evaluation of sleep maintenance insomnia in PD. While continuous positive airway pressure (CPAP) has been associated with improved sleep quality in PD (Kaminska et al., 2018), there are challenges to applying CPAP in PD (Terzaghi et al., 2017; see Chapter 8 for more information on sleep disordered breathing in PD).

Among PD patients reporting poor sleep, greater amounts of sleep fragmentation have been seen on polysomnography in some studies (Norlinah et al., 2009).

Consequences and complications

Insomnia is cited as being the most bothersome symptom among at least 10% of advanced PD patients (Politis et al., 2010). Insomnia in PD is associated with a significantly worse quality of life (Avidan et al., 2013; Barone et al., 2009; Duncan et al., 2014; Forsaa, Larsen, Wentzel-Larsen, Herlofson, & Alves, 2008; Kasten et al., 2012; Shearer, Green, Counsell, & Zajicek, 2012). PD patients with insomnia are more likely to have more severe motor and nonmotor manifestations as compared with PD patients without insomnia. The directionality of this relationship is unclear. In other words, whether the insomnia contributes to the other nonmotor features, whether the other nonmotor features cause or exacerbate the insomnia, or both is not well understood. Another possibility is that all these nonmotor features are manifestations of underlying neurodegeneration (rather than necessarily being causes or consequences of each other). With that in mind, it is of note that PD patients with insomnia are more likely to suffer from depression and dysautonomia (Chung et al., 2013; Gjerstad et al., 2007; Tholfsen et al., 2017). Being aware of these comorbidities may improve their detection and management; whether the latter in turn improves outcomes of each remains to be seen.

Studies on the daytime consequences of insomnia in PD suggest that in at least a subset of patients, daytime sleepiness is not objectively increased (Chung et al., 2013). Having said, subjective excessive daytime sleepiness is present in many patients who report subjective sleep maintenance insomnia (Tholfsen et al., 2017), and several other adverse daytime consequences of insomnia may manifest even in the absence of daytime sleepiness, such as fatigue and difficulty concentrating (based on data from the general population).

Management

There is limited evidence to guide the treatment of sleep maintenance insomnia in PD. The Movement Disorders Society (MDS) evidence-based medicine review on treatments of nonmotor symptoms of PD rated eszopiclone and 3—5 mg of melatonin as possibly useful (Seppi et al., 2019). Trials for eszopiclone for PD insomnia have been limited by small sample sizes. One 6-week trial in 30 patients showed significantly reduced number of awakenings, subjective sleep quality, and overall improvement on the physician-rated clinical global impression scale, although no significant improvement in the primary outcome of TST was found (Menza et al., 2010). If a trial of eszopiclone for PD insomnia is initiated, it is important to keep in mind that in older adults, use of eszopiclone and other sedative hypnotics should be limited to brief treatment trials (Schutte-Rodin, Broch, Buysse, Dorsey, & Sateia, 2008).

As for melatonin, there are also no clear data to guide the dose of melatonin that best weighs efficacy versus side effects. The MDS task force indicated that 3—5 mg dose carries acceptable risk without the need for specialized monitoring (Seppi et al., 2019) and concluded that the 50 mg dose is considered investigational with insufficient evidence to make conclusions about safety. The 50 mg dose of melatonin for insomnia in PD was studied in a 10-week crossover study in 40 patients who completed the trial. Outcome measures included nocturnal activity monitoring with actigraphy as well as questionnaires. 50 mg of melatonin at bedtime significantly improved total nighttime sleep duration as measured by actigraphy compared with placebo and 5 mg (Dowling et al., 2005), but only by 10 minutes. The clinical significance of this finding is unclear.

As for the effect of PD medications on sleep maintenance, controlled-release levodopa was rated as investigational by the MDS task force (Seppi et al., 2019). In a one-night open-label study, controlled-release carbidopa/levodopa 50/200 mg was associated with a mean of 15 minutes less of WASO on polysomnography as compared with those who did not take dopaminergic medications that night (Wailke, Herzog, Witt, Deuschl, & Volkmann, 2011). While this difference was statistically significant, the clinical significance of 15 minutes less of WASO is not clear. Rotigotine, which has been tested in an open-label study for insomnia in PD (Trenkwalder et al., 2011), was rated as possibly useful by the task force, with acceptable risk without the need for specialized monitoring (Seppi et al., 2019).

Sodium oxybate as a treatment for insomnia in PD was first examined in an open-label study (Ondo et al., 2008) and then in a small pilot randomized controlled trial in 12 patients (Buchele et al., 2018). Sodium oxybate was associated with improved subjective sleep quality and with polysomnographically measured slow wave sleep duration. Side effects include parasomnia in one patient and new onset sleep apnea in two patients. Given safety concerns, additional studies are needed before sodium oxybate could be considered a treatment for insomnia in PD.

Benzodiazepines are associated with increased risk of falls and may exacerbate daytime sleepiness and cognitive dysfunction in older adults (Frank, 2014). Having said that, in some instances, they may be necessary in PD, such as for treatment of comorbid severe REM sleep behavior disorder (RBD) (see Chapter 5 for more on REM sleep behavior disorder). In those cases, anecdotal evidence indicates they can help sleep onset and maintenance insomnia as well. Given the risks of benzodiazepines though (Frank, 2014), they should be used only sparingly for treatment of insomnia in PD.

When comorbidities are present in PD patients with insomnia, rationale selection of medications is advised, to help treat not only the insomnia but also these comorbidities (Table 2.2).

Table 2.2 Rationale use of pharmacotherapy to treat disorders comorbid with insomnia in Parkinson's disorder (PD).

Drug class	Comments	Adverse event considerations
Antidepressants	Sedating antidepressants such as nortriptyline or sertraline may be useful for both depression and/or anxiety and may help insomnia in PD	Selective serotonin reuptake inhibitors, selective serotonin-norepinephrine reuptake inhibitors may exacerbate both restless legs syndrome (RLS) and REM sleep behavior disorder (RBD).
Benzodiazepines	Useful for comorbid refractory RLS (short-acting) and RBD (long-acting)	Increased risk of falling and cognitive dysfunction
Nuplazid	May be useful for sleep problems in the setting of nocturnal psychosis	Limited data available on effect of nuplazid on sleep
Antipsychotics	Antipsychotics with low potency at dopamine receptors (quetiapine, clozapine) may be useful for very select cases in which there are sleep problems in the setting of nocturnal psychosis	Limited data available on utility for nocturnal psychosis/sleep problems. Antipsychotics are associated with increased mortality and with worsening parkinsonism. Quetiapine is not appropriate for isolated sleep onset insomnia but only when other comorbidities are being targeted as well

For example, depression and anxiety are often comorbid with insomnia in PD. In some clinical trials for depression and anxiety treatment in PD, where sleep has been included as a secondary outcome, improvements in sleep were reported, including for nortriptyline (Dobkin et al., 2011; Menza et al., 2009) and venlafaxine (Richard et al., 2012). While mirtazapine has not been studied in PD for treatment of depression or insomnia, data from the general older adult population may suggest that in some instances it may be considered for PD patients with insomnia and depression and/or anxiety. The same applies for trazodone. Having said that, there are factors in PD beyond the general older adult population that require specific consideration. Namely, exacerbation of some sleep disorders by antidepressants, including RLS and RBD, may be particularly likely to occur in PD (see Chapter 3 for more information regarding the contribution of mood and anxiety disorders to insomnia in PD).

Like benzodiazepines, antipsychotic use in PD should be limited only to clearly indicated cases. This is especially true given the adverse event profile of antipsychotics in older adults in general and in PD in specific (Weintraub et al., 2017). Antipsychotic use has been associated with increased mortality in PD (Weintraub et al., 2016), although causality cannot necessarily be inferred from existing data. In instances where nocturnal psychosis requires treatment with antipsychotic agents, their sedating properties may be useful to help with insomnia as well. Quetiapine and clozaril are the two antipsychotics least likely to exacerbate parkinsonism in PD; these were rated as possibly and clinically useful, respectively, for treatment of psychosis in PD by the MDS task force (Seppi et al., 2019; see Chapter 4 for more information on the contribution of psychosis to nocturnal symptoms in PD and its management).

Finally, in terms of behavioral interventions to treat sleep problems in PD, preliminary data from pilot studies indicate that exercise might improve nighttime sleep in PD (Coe et al., 2018; Silva-Batista et al., 2017). In a 24-week randomized trial of resistance exercise in 29 PD patients with PD compared with 36 controls, subjective assessment of nighttime sleep and daytime sleepiness occurred via nonvalidated questionnaires, and actigraphy was also recorded. Significant decreases in nocturnal mobility (an indirect measure that could indicate increased nighttime sleep) were found after the exercise intervention and also after the control intervention (Coe et al., 2018). In a 12-week randomized, controlled trial 11 PD subjects were randomized to a progressive resistance training program and 11 to a nonexercise group. Subjective nighttime sleep, as assessed with the Pittsburgh Sleep Quality Index questionnaire, significantly improved in the intervention arm compared with the control arm (Silva-Batista et al., 2017). Additional data are needed, but results are encouraging that exercise can improve nighttime sleep in PD.

Illustrative case in context

In the case presented, the patient reports sleep fragmentation and prolonged nocturnal awakenings. There are several potential contributing factors including motor problems, nocturia, and daytime napping. Addressing each of these individually would be important to treating his insomnia. For example, a bedtime or overnight dose of levodopa would be indicated. Urologic evaluation would be appropriate (see Chapter 10 for more information on nocturia in PD and its management). Finally, limiting daytime naps would help as well. If these interventions are not sufficient, initiation of a medication such as trazodone would be appropriate. Starting at the lowest dose of 25 mg at bedtime and increasing gradually as needed would be prudent. Risks of oversedation and morning grogginess should be discussed (and in males, priapism).

References

American Academy of Sleep Medicine. (2014). *International classification of sleep disorders* (3rd ed.). Darien, IL: American Academy of Sleep Medicine.

Avidan, A., Hays, R. D., Diaz, N., Bordelon, Y., Thompson, A. W., Vassar, S. D., et al. (2013). Associations of sleep disturbance symptoms with health-related quality of life in Parkinson's disease. *The Journal of Neuropsychiatry and Clinical Neurosciences, 25*(4), 319—326.

Barone, P., Antonini, A., Colosimo, C., Marconi, R., Morgante, L., Avarello, T. P., et al. (2009). The PRIAMO study: A multicenter assessment of nonmotor symptoms and their impact on quality of life in Parkinson's disease. *Movement Disorders: Official Journal of the Movement Disorder Society, 24*(11), 1641—1649.

Barone, P., Poewe, W., Albrecht, S., Debieuvre, C., Massey, D., Rascol, O., et al. (2010). Pramipexole for the treatment of depressive symptoms in patients with Parkinson's disease: A randomised, double-blind, placebo-controlled trial. *Lancet Neurology, 9*(6), 573—580.

Buchele, F., Hackius, M., Schreglmann, S. R., Omlor, W., Werth, E., Maric, A., et al. (2018). Sodium oxybate for excessive daytime sleepiness and sleep disturbance in Parkinson disease: A randomized clinical trial. *JAMA Neurology, 75*(1), 114—118.

Chahine, L. M., Daley, J., Horn, S., Duda, J. E., Colcher, A., Hurtig, H., et al. (2013). Association between dopaminergic medications and nocturnal sleep in early-stage Parkinson's disease. *Parkinsonism & Related Disorders, 19*(10), 859—863.

Chung, S., Bohnen, N. I., Albin, R. L., Frey, K. A., Muller, M. L., & Chervin, R. D. (2013). Insomnia and sleepiness in Parkinson disease: Associations with symptoms and comorbidities. *Journal of Clinical Sleep Medicine: Official Publication of the American Academy of Sleep Medicine, 9*(11), 1131—1137.

Coe, S., Franssen, M., Collett, J., Boyle, D., Meaney, A., Chantry, R., et al. (2018). Physical activity, fatigue, and sleep in people with Parkinson's disease: A secondary per protocol analysis from an intervention trial. *Parkinson's Disease, 2018*, 1517807.

Dobkin, R. D., Menza, M., Bienfait, K. L., Gara, M., Marin, H., Mark, M. H., et al. (2011). Depression in Parkinson's disease: Symptom improvement and residual symptoms after acute pharmacologic management. *The American Journal of Geriatric Psychiatry: Official Journal of the American Association for Geriatric Psychiatry, 19*(3), 222—229.

Dowling, G. A., Mastick, J., Colling, E., Carter, J. H., Singer, C. M., & Aminoff, M. J. (2005). Melatonin for sleep disturbances in Parkinson's disease. *Sleep Medicine, 6*(5), 459—466.

Duncan, G. W., Khoo, T. K., Yarnall, A. J., O'Brien, J. T., Coleman, S. Y., Brooks, D. J., et al. (2014). Health-related quality of life in early Parkinson's disease: The impact of nonmotor symptoms. *Movement Disorders: Official Journal of the Movement Disorder Society, 29*(2), 195—202.

Forsaa, E. B., Larsen, J. P., Wentzel-Larsen, T., Herlofson, K., & Alves, G. (2008). Predictors and course of health-related quality of life in Parkinson's disease. *Movement Disorders: Official Journal of the Movement Disorder Society, 23*(10), 1420−1427.

Frank, C. (2014). Pharmacologic treatment of depression in the elderly. *Canadian Family Physician Medecin De Famille Canadien, 60*(2), 121−126.

Gjerstad, M. D., Wentzel-Larsen, T., Aarsland, D., & Larsen, J. P. (2007). Insomnia in Parkinson's disease: Frequency and progression over time. *Journal of Neurology, Neurosurgery & Psychiatry, 78*(5), 476−479.

Gomez-Esteban, J. C., Zarranz, J. J., Lezcano, E., Velasco, F., Ciordia, R., Rouco, I., et al. (2006). Sleep complaints and their relation with drug treatment in patients suffering from Parkinson's disease. *Movement Disorders: Official Journal of the Movement Disorder Society, 21*(7), 983−988.

Jongwanasiri, S., Prayoonwiwat, N., Pisarnpong, A., Srivanitchapoom, P., & Chotinaiwattarakul, W. (2014). Evaluation of sleep disorders in Parkinson's disease: A comparison between physician diagnosis and self-administered questionnaires. *Journal of the Medical Association of Thailand = Chotmaihet Thangphaet, 97*(Suppl. 3), S68−S77.

Kaminska, M., Mery, V. P., Lafontaine, A. L., Robinson, A., Benedetti, A., Gros, P., et al. (2018). Change in cognition and other non-motor symptoms with obstructive sleep apnea treatment in Parkinson disease. *Journal of Clinical Sleep Medicine: Official Publication of the American Academy of Sleep Medicine, 14*(5), 819−828.

Kasten, M., Kertelge, L., Tadic, V., Bruggemann, N., Schmidt, A., van der Vegt, J., et al. (2012). Depression and quality of life in monogenic compared to idiopathic, early-onset Parkinson's disease. *Movement Disorders: Official Journal of the Movement Disorder Society, 27*(6), 754−759.

Louter, M., van Sloun, R. J., Pevernagie, D. A., Arends, J. B., Cluitmans, P. J., Bloem, B. R., et al. (2013). Subjectively impaired bed mobility in Parkinson disease affects sleep efficiency. *Sleep Medicine, 14*(7), 668−674.

Lyons, K. E., Friedman, J. H., Hermanowicz, N., Isaacson, S. H., Hauser, R. A., Hersh, B. P., et al. (2010). Orally disintegrating selegiline in Parkinson patients with dopamine agonist-related adverse effects. *Clinical Neuropharmacology, 33*(1), 5−10.

Menza, M., Dobkin, R. D., Marin, H., Gara, M., Bienfait, K., Dicke, A., et al. (2010). Treatment of insomnia in Parkinson's disease: A controlled trial of eszopiclone and placebo. *Movement Disorders: Official Journal of the Movement Disorder Society, 25*(11), 1708−1714.

Menza, M., Dobkin, R. D., Marin, H., Mark, M. H., Gara, M., Buyske, S., et al. (2009). A controlled trial of antidepressants in patients with Parkinson disease and depression. *Neurology, 72*(10), 886−892.

Norlinah, M. I., Afidah, K. N., Noradina, A. T., Shamsul, A. S., Hamidon, B. B., Sahathevan, R., et al. (2009). Sleep disturbances in Malaysian patients with Parkinson's disease using polysomnography and PDSS. *Parkinsonism & Related Disorders, 15*(9), 670−674.

Ondo, W. G., Perkins, T., Swick, T., Hull, K. L., Jr., Jimenez, J. E., Garris, T. S., et al. (2008). Sodium oxybate for excessive daytime sleepiness in Parkinson disease: An open-label polysomnographic study. *Archives of Neurology, 65*(10), 1337−1340.

Politis, M., Wu, K., Molloy, S., G Bain, P., Chaudhuri, K. R., & Piccini, P. (2010). Parkinson's disease symptoms: The patient's perspective. *Movement Disorders: Official Journal of the Movement Disorder Society, 25*(11), 1646−1651.

Porter, B., Macfarlane, R., & Walker, R. (2008). The frequency and nature of sleep disorders in a community-based population of patients with Parkinson's disease. *European Journal of Neurology: The Official Journal of the European Federation of Neurological Societies, 15*(1), 50–54.

Richard, I. H., McDermott, M. P., Kurlan, R., Lyness, J. M., Como, P. G., Pearson, N., et al. (2012). A randomized, double-blind, placebo-controlled trial of antidepressants in Parkinson disease. *Neurology, 78*(16), 1229–1236.

Schutte-Rodin, S., Broch, L., Buysse, D., Dorsey, C., & Sateia, M. (2008). Clinical guideline for the evaluation and management of chronic insomnia in adults. *Journal of Clinical Sleep Medicine: Official Publication of the American Academy of Sleep Medicine, 4*(5), 487–504.

Seppi, K., Ray Chaudhuri, K., Coelho, M., Fox, S. H., Katzenschlager, R., Perez Lloret, S., et al. (2019). Update on treatments for nonmotor symptoms of Parkinson's disease-an evidence-based medicine review. *Movement Disorders: Official Journal of the Movement Disorder Society, 34*(2), 180–198.

Shearer, J., Green, C., Counsell, C. E., & Zajicek, J. P. (2012). The impact of motor and non motor symptoms on health state values in newly diagnosed idiopathic Parkinson's disease. *Journal of Neurology, 259*(3), 462–468.

Silva-Batista, C., de Brito, L. C., Corcos, D. M., Roschel, H., de Mello, M. T., Piemonte, M. E. P., et al. (2017). Resistance training improves sleep quality in subjects with moderate Parkinson's disease. *The Journal of Strength & Conditioning Research, 31*(8), 2270–2277.

Stack, E. L., & Ashburn, A. M. (2006). Impaired bed mobility and disordered sleep in Parkinson's disease. *Movement Disorders: Official Journal of the Movement Disorder Society, 21*(9), 1340–1342.

Stern, M., Roffwarg, H., & Duvoisin, R. (1968). The parkinsonian tremor in sleep. *The Journal of Nervous and Mental Disease, 147*(2), 202–210.

Suzuki, K., Miyamoto, M., Miyamoto, T., Okuma, Y., Hattori, N., Kamei, S., et al. (2009). Correlation between depressive symptoms and nocturnal disturbances in Japanese patients with Parkinson's disease. *Parkinsonism & Related Disorders, 15*(1), 15–19.

Terzaghi, M., Spelta, L., Minafra, B., Rustioni, V., Zangaglia, R., Pacchetti, C., et al. (2017). Treating sleep apnea in Parkinson's disease with C-PAP: Feasibility concerns and effects on cognition and alertness. *Sleep Medicine, 33*, 114–118.

Tholfsen, L. K., Larsen, J. P., Schulz, J., Tysnes, O. B., & Gjerstad, M. D. (2017). Changes in insomnia subtypes in early Parkinson disease. *Neurology, 88*(4), 352–358.

Trenkwalder, C., Kies, B., Rudzinska, M., Fine, J., Nikl, J., Honczarenko, K., et al. (2011). Rotigotine effects on early morning motor function and sleep in Parkinson's disease: A double-blind, randomized, placebo-controlled study (RECOVER). *Movement Disorders: Official Journal of the Movement Disorder Society, 26*(1), 90–99.

Tse, W., Liu, Y., Barthlen, G. M., Halbig, T. D., Tolgyesi, S. V., Gracies, J. M., et al. (2005). Clinical usefulness of the Parkinson's disease sleep scale. *Parkinsonism & Related Disorders, 11*(5), 317–321.

Verbaan, D., van Rooden, S. M., Visser, M., Marinus, J., & van Hilten, J. J. (2008). Nighttime sleep problems and daytime sleepiness in Parkinson's disease. *Movement Disorders: Official Journal of the Movement Disorder Society, 23*(1), 35–41.

Wailke, S., Herzog, J., Witt, K., Deuschl, G., & Volkmann, J. (2011). Effect of controlled-release levodopa on the microstructure of sleep in Parkinson's disease. *European Journal of Neurology: The Official Journal of the European Federation of Neurological Societies, 18*(4), 590–596.

Weintraub, D., Chiang, C., Kim, H. M., Wilkinson, J., Marras, C., Stanislawski, B., et al. (2016). Association of antipsychotic use with mortality risk in patients with Parkinson disease. *JAMA Neurology, 73*(5), 535−541.

Weintraub, D., Chiang, C., Kim, H. M., Wilkinson, J., Marras, C., Stanislawski, B., et al. (2017). Antipsychotic use and physical morbidity in Parkinson disease. *The American Journal of Geriatric Psychiatry: Official Journal of the American Association for Geriatric Psychiatry, 25*(7), 697−705.

Yong, M. H., Fook-Chong, S., Pavanni, R., Lim, L. L., & Tan, E. K. (2011). Case control polysomnographic studies of sleep disorders in Parkinson's disease. *PLoS One, 6*(7), e22511.

Zhou, C. Q., Zhang, J. W., Wang, M., & Peng, G. G. (2014). Meta-analysis of the efficacy and safety of long-acting non-ergot dopamine agonists in Parkinson's disease. *Journal of Clinical Neuroscience: Official Journal of the Neurosurgical Society of Australasia, 21*(7), 1094−1101.

Contribution of mood and anxiety disorders to sleep problems

Illustrative case

A 52-year-old woman with Parkinson's disease (PD) of 3 years' duration reports several sleep complaints. She has trouble falling asleep and attributes this to her "thoughts running" and not being able to "turn off" her mind. Once she finally does get to sleep, she sleeps in bouts of 2–3 hours. On some nights, she wakes up with a sense of fear and panic, with associated sweating and palpitations. These episodes are not necessarily associated with nightmares or other triggers that she can identify. Most mornings, she wakes up at 4–5 a.m. and cannot get back to sleep. She is very frustrated with these sleep problems; she is tired during the day and having difficulty concentrating. She also reports feeling down and depressed during the day, worries "all the time about everything," and has occasional episodes of panic attacks during the day as well. On directed questioning, her motor symptoms are generally well controlled on carbidopa/levodopa 25/100 mg, one tablet every 4 hours, along with ropinirole extended release, 6 mg at bedtime. However, sometimes when she is late taking her dose, she does get a sense of chest pressure and an anxious feeling.

Overview

Definition

To understand the contribution of mood and anxiety disorders to sleep problems in PD requires a basic understanding of the diagnostic criteria for these disorders and nuances in this regard in PD.

In the general population, according to the Diagnostic and Statistical Manual (DSM), Fifth Edition, the diagnosis of depression is based on the presence of depressed mood most of the day nearly every day, associated with other symptoms such as weight loss or weight gait, fatigue, cognitive changes, thoughts of death, and having an impact on function (American Psychiatric Association, 2013). Diagnosis of depression in PD requires the accounting for the broad spectrum of manifestations of depression in PD, the overlap with other disorders and symptoms that are often

Disorders of Sleep and Wakefulness in Parkinson's Disease. https://doi.org/10.1016/B978-0-323-67374-7.00003-1

comorbid with PD, and the relationship between psychiatric symptoms, motor problems, and their treatment (Marsh, McDonald, Cummings, Ravina, & NINDS/NIMH Work Group on Depression and Parkinson's Disease, 2006). Indeed, the relationship between depression and sleep problems in PD is a good example of this complexity. Sleep symptoms (insomnia or hypersomnia) are considered a core symptom in the diagnostic criteria for depression (American Psychiatric Association, 2013) in the general population, but nondepressed PD patients often also suffer from sleep problems (Marsh et al., 2006).

Guidance on the diagnostic criteria for depression in PD has been put forth that accounts for nuances in relation to diagnosing mood disorders in PD (Marsh et al., 2006). The general recommendation is to apply the criteria put forth in the DSM (American Psychiatric Association, 2013), but with some modifications. An inclusive approach has been recommended whereby the presence of symptoms is considered inclusively regardless of their presumed etiology. Distinguishing between primary apathy and dementia, where possible, is suggested.

As for anxiety disorders, the DSM-5 includes five major types: generalized anxiety disorder, obsessive compulsive disorder, panic disorder, posttraumatic stress disorder (PTSD), and social phobia (American Psychiatric Association, 2013). Of relevance to sleep problems in PD are mainly generalized anxiety, panic disorder, and PTSD. The core diagnostic criterion for generalized anxiety involves excessive anxiety and worry, with difficulty controlling the worry and an impact on function. As for panic disorder, the core criteria include recurrent panic attacks marked by symptoms such as palpitations, dyspnea, or sweating, not accounted for by other medical problems.

Epidemiology

Depression is common in PD (Marsh et al., 2006). About 35% of PD patients have clinically relevant depressive symptomatology (Reijnders, Ehrt, Weber, Aarsland, & Leentjens, 2008), and 19% meet DSM-IV criteria for depression based on semistructured interview. In the inpatient setting, prevalence of depression in PD is as high as 50%.

Regarding the prevalence of anxiety disorders, questionnaire-based studies indicate that anxiety is more common and more severe in PD compared with age- and sex-matched controls (Menza & Mark, 1994). Anxiety symptoms occur in 25%−40% of PD patients (Dissanayaka et al., 2010; Leentjens et al., 2008; Pontone et al., 2009), even in early PD (Khoo et al., 2013). Up to one-third meet criteria for panic disorder (Leentjens et al., 2008; Pontone et al., 2009), and generalized anxiety disorder occurs in 3%−11% (Dissanayaka et al., 2010; Leentjens et al., 2008). Robust data on the prevalence of nocturnal panic in PD are lacking.

Depression and anxiety symptoms are often comorbid in PD (Pontone et al., 2009); 92% of PD patients with a diagnosis of an anxiety disorder had depression symptoms and 67% of patients with depression had symptoms of anxiety (Menza, Robertson-Hoffman, & Bonapace, 1993).

As for the epidemiology of the comorbidity of sleep and depression and/or anxiety in PD, several questionnaire-based studies consistently show a moderate to strong correlation between measures of sleep, depression, and/or anxiety symptoms (Kay, Tanner, & Bowers, 2018; Shafazand et al., 2017; Suzuki et al., 2009). The relationship is bidirectional, as highlighted throughout this chapter. In one of the few studies examining the relationship between depression, anxiety, and sleep disturbances in PD longitudinally, data from 361 newly diagnosed PD patients (within 2 years of diagnosis) who were untreated for PD at baseline were included (Rutten et al., 2017). Anxiety was assessed with the State Trait Anxiety Inventory (STAI), depression with the 15-item Geriatric Depression Scale and sleep with an item from the Movement Disorders Society Unified Parkinson's Disease Rating scales that asks: "Over the past week have you had trouble going to sleep at night or staying asleep through the night? Consider how rested you felt after waking up in the morning". A response of two or more (on a 0—4 scale) was considered to indicate insomnia. 23% of the cohort had insomnia at baseline, 3.6% had clinically relevant anxiety and 14% had depression. The presence of anxiety and depression at baseline both predicted presence of insomnia at 6-month follow-up, and on the other hand, the presence of insomnia at baseline predicted higher STAI state score on follow-up (but not trait anxiety scores or higher depression scores) (Rutten et al., 2017).

Etiology and differential diagnosis

A common neurobiologic basis, namely abnormalities in monoaminergic and cholinergic transmission, may account at least in part for the common comorbidity of sleep problems, anxiety, and depression in PD. On the other hand, depression and anxiety may manifest with sleep problems in PD. In turn, sleep problems may contribute to depression and anxiety.

As mentioned, the relationship between depression and insomnia in PD is likely bidirectional. PD patients with depression are more likely to have poor sleep (Chung et al., 2013; Gjerstad, Wentzel-Larsen, Aarsland, & Larsen, 2007; Porter, Macfarlane, & Walker, 2008; Verbaan, van Rooden, Visser, Marinus, & van Hilten, 2008; Yong, Fook-Chong, Pavanni, Lim, & Tan, 2011; Yu et al., 2013), and PD patients with insomnia are more likely to have depression (Suzuki et al., 2009). One analysis of 419 PD patients, in which subjective sleep quality was assessed with the SCOPA-SLEEP scale, demonstrated that depression symptoms account for 21% of the variance in poor nighttime sleep symptoms (Verbaan et al., 2008). As for the relationship between anxiety and sleep in PD, one study found that PD patients with anxiety reported less-refreshing sleep, but anxiety did not contribute to the overall variance in sleep quality, which was largely accounted for by PD disease severity, especially in relation to off/on phenomena (Menza & Rosen, 1995). Also as mentioned, there are few data on panic disorder in PD and its contribution to sleep problems. In the general population, over 60% of patients with panic disorder report poor subjective sleep, even in the absence of identified nocturnal panic attacks. In those with panic disorder with nocturnal panic attacks, the prevalence of poor subjective sleep is over 90% (Singareddy & Uhde, 2009).

In approaching the diagnosis and management of nocturnal depression and anxiety symptoms, it is important to determine to what degree these are a manifestation of wearing off of dopaminergic medications (Marsh et al., 2006). This is a critical distinction because if symptoms of panic, anxiety, and/or depression occur strictly in the "off" state, when the effects of dopaminergic medications have worn off (with neutral or even euphoric mood in the "on" state) (Racette et al., 2002), this requires management largely to target wearing off, rather than just treatments targeted at the depression and anxiety symptoms per se. Indeed, motor fluctuations are a risk factor for panic symptoms and anxiety in PD (Dissanayaka et al., 2010; Pontone et al., 2009; Vazquez, Jimenez-Jimenez, Garcia-Ruiz, & Garcia-Urra, 1993), and anxiety, panic, and depression are common nonmotor manifestations of wearing off (Racette et al., 2002; Vazquez et al., 1993).

Consequences and complications

Mood and anxiety disorders in PD could be associated with sleep initiation insomnia (see Chapter 1), sleep maintenance insomnia (see Chapter 2), and early-morning awakenings. In a study of 50 PD subjective and 48 age- and sex-matched controls, the relationship of subjective total sleep time as reported on the Pittsburgh Sleep Quality Index (PSQI) to depression symptoms as measured on the Beck Depression Inventory (BDI) was assessed. Shorter total sleep time and insomnia severity were associated with severity of depression symptoms on the BDI-II (Kay et al., 2018).

In a study of 188 PD patients with varying disease severity and duration, sleep was assessed with the Parkinson's' Disease Sleep Scale (PDSS) and depression with the Zung Self-rating Depression Scale (Suzuki et al., 2009). PDSS score was a significant predictor of depression even after adjusting for potential confounders. Among depressed patients, the most common sleep symptoms reported were sleep fragmentation, daytime sleepiness, dystonia, and tremor (Suzuki et al., 2009). In a cohort of earlier PD, presence of both depression and anxiety symptoms predicted insomnia on follow-up (Rutten et al., 2017).

As for objective sleep measures, in a small study examining sleep in 8 PD patients with depression compared with 18 PD without depression (Kostic, Susic, Przedborski, & Sternic, 1991), shortened latency to rapid eye movement (REM) sleep ($\leq$65 minutes) was more common in depressed patients compared with nondepressed patients. Shortened REM latency is a common and relatively specific finding in depression in the general population, and the findings of this study likely reflect the idea that depression affects sleep in PD the same way it affects sleep in the general population. Whether there are other consequences of this REM latency abnormality in PD patients per se is not clear. One interesting possibility is that depression could mediate the expression of RBD in PD (see Chapter 7 for more on RBD in PD).

In turn, sleep problems may exacerbate depression and anxiety. In a study of 66 PD patients with moderate PD (Shafazand et al., 2017), insomnia was assessed with the Athens Insomnia Scale, sleep quality with the PSQI, sleep symptoms with the PDSS, and depression with the BDI-II. Among PD patients reporting insomnia, BDI-II scores were significantly higher compared with those without insomnia (Shafazand et al., 2017). Another study in 361 PD patients with early PD also demonstrated that presence of insomnia was associated with higher anxiety scores on follow-up (Rutten et al., 2017).

Management

In the setting of a diagnosable mood or anxiety disorder in PD, treatments targeting that underlying disorder may help the comorbid sleep problems. Where possible, the rationale use of medications to treat multiple comorbidities in PD would be optimal. The Movement Disorders Society has issued an evidence-based review of nonmotor symptoms in PD, which classifies several medications as efficacious or likely efficacious for treatment of depression in PD, including pramipexole, nortriptyline and desipramine, and venlafaxine. In randomized controlled trials of nortriptyline, paroxetine, and venlafaxine for depression in PD, insomnia was studied as a secondary outcome (Dobkin et al., 2011; Menza et al., 2009; Richard et al., 2012). Those studies indicate that treating depression in PD is associated with an improvement in symptoms of poor sleep. While data supporting the efficacy of sertraline and mirtazapine in PD are limited, in some instances in PD patients with the symptom complex of sleep onset and maintenance insomnia, depression, and anxiety, anecdotal evidence and data from the general older adult population suggest these sedating antidepressants may be considered as well. When antidepressants are used in PD, monitoring for worsening of RBD or RLS is necessary.

In instances where symptoms of depression and anxiety are resulting from wearing off of dopaminergic medication, the treatment strategy is mainly to optimize the dopaminergic medication regimen and to address the "wearing off" of PD medications. In some cases, addition of a controlled-release formulation of levodopa or an extended-release formulation of a dopamine agonist can help. Indeed, rotigotine has been associated with improved sleep quality in PD.

When nocturnal anxiety and panic symptoms cannot be mitigated with adjustment of dopaminergic medications and/or antidepressants, the cautious and targeted use of benzodiazepines may be indicated in select cases (Chaudhuri, 2003). This is especially true when other disorders that benefit from benzodiazepine treatment, namely REM sleep behavior disorder, are present.

Illustrative case in context

In the case presented, the patient is a 52-year-old woman with sleep initiation and sleep maintenance insomnia as well as early-morning awakening. Her history indicates she is suffering from anxiety, depression, and panic attacks. Cognitive-behavioral interventions may be useful to help with the contribution of anxiety to her sleep initiation insomnia. She might also benefit from a sedating antidepressant such as sertraline or mirtazapine, to be taken at bedtime. This may help both her nocturnal symptoms as well as treat her underlying depression and panic disorder. There is possibly a component of nonmotor wearing off manifesting with anxiety and panic, and adding a bedtime dose of controlled-release levodopa, as well as possibly overnight dosing of carbidopa/levodopa immediate release as needed would be useful. Since her panic attacks are not common, if she has residual occasional attacks after all these interventions, short-acting benzodiazepines could be considered, to be used sparingly only when she has significant discomfort from a panic attack.

References

American Psychiatric Association. (2013). *Diagnostic and statistical manual of mental disorders* (5th ed.). Arlington, VA: American Psychiatric Publishing.

Chaudhuri, K. R. (2003). Nocturnal symptom complex in PD and its management. *Neurology, 61*(6 Suppl. 3), S17−S23.

Chung, S., Bohnen, N. I., Albin, R. L., Frey, K. A., Muller, M. L., & Chervin, R. D. (2013). Insomnia and sleepiness in Parkinson disease: Associations with symptoms and comorbidities. *Journal of Clinical Sleep Medicine: Official Publication of the American Academy of Sleep Medicine, 9*(11), 1131−1137.

Dissanayaka, N. N., Sellbach, A., Matheson, S., O'Sullivan, J. D., Silburn, P. A., Byrne, G. J., et al. (2010). Anxiety disorders in Parkinson's disease: Prevalence and risk factors. *Movement Disorders: Official Journal of the Movement Disorder Society, 25*(7), 838−845.

Dobkin, R. D., Menza, M., Bienfait, K. L., Gara, M., Marin, H., Mark, M. H., et al. (2011). Depression in Parkinson's disease: Symptom improvement and residual symptoms after acute pharmacologic management. *American Journal of Geriatric Psychiatry: Official Journal of the American Association for Geriatric Psychiatry, 19*(3), 222−229.

Gjerstad, M. D., Wentzel-Larsen, T., Aarsland, D., & Larsen, J. P. (2007). Insomnia in Parkinson's disease: Frequency and progression over time. *Journal of Neurology, Neurosurgery & Psychiatry, 78*(5), 476−479.

Kay, D. B., Tanner, J. J., & Bowers, D. (2018). Sleep disturbances and depression severity in patients with Parkinson's disease. *Brain and Behavior, 8*(6), e00967.

Khoo, T. K., Yarnall, A. J., Duncan, G. W., Coleman, S., O'Brien, J. T., Brooks, D. J., et al. (2013). The spectrum of nonmotor symptoms in early Parkinson disease. *Neurology, 80*(3), 276−281.

Kostic, V. S., Susic, V., Przedborski, S., & Sternic, N. (1991). Sleep EEG in depressed and nondepressed patients with Parkinson's disease. *Journal of Neuropsychiatry and Clinical Neurosciences, 3*(2), 176−179.

Leentjens, A. F., Dujardin, K., Marsh, L., Martinez-Martin, P., Richard, I. H., Starkstein, S. E., et al. (2008). Anxiety rating scales in Parkinson's disease: Critique and recommendations. *Movement Disorders: Official Journal of the Movement Disorder Society, 23*(14), 2015−2025.

Marsh, L., McDonald, W. M., Cummings, J., Ravina, B., & NINDS/NIMH Work Group on Depression and Parkinson's Disease. (2006). Provisional diagnostic criteria for depression in Parkinson's disease: Report of an NINDS/NIMH work group. *Movement Disorders: Official Journal of the Movement Disorder Society, 21*(2), 148−158.

Menza, M. A., & Mark, M. H. (1994). Parkinson's disease and depression: The relationship to disability and personality. *Journal of Neuropsychiatry and Clinical Neurosciences, 6*(2), 165−169.

Menza, M. A., & Rosen, R. C. (1995). Sleep in Parkinson's disease. The role of depression and anxiety. *Psychosomatics, 36*(3), 262−266.

Menza, M., Dobkin, R. D., Marin, H., Mark, M. H., Gara, M., Buyske, S., et al. (2009). A controlled trial of antidepressants in patients with Parkinson disease and depression. *Neurology, 72*(10), 886−892.

Menza, M. A., Robertson-Hoffman, D. E., & Bonapace, A. S. (1993). Parkinson's disease and anxiety: Comorbidity with depression. *Biological Psychiatry, 34*(7), 465−470.

Pontone, G. M., Williams, J. R., Anderson, K. E., Chase, G., Goldstein, S. A., Grill, S., et al. (2009). Prevalence of anxiety disorders and anxiety subtypes in patients with Parkinson's disease. *Movement Disorders: Official Journal of the Movement Disorder Society, 24*(9), 1333−1338.

Porter, B., Macfarlane, R., & Walker, R. (2008). The frequency and nature of sleep disorders in a community-based population of patients with Parkinson's disease. *European Journal of Neurology: The Official Journal of the European Federation of Neurological Societies, 15*(1), 50−54.

Racette, B. A., Hartlein, J. M., Hershey, T., Mink, J. W., Perlmutter, J. S., & Black, K. J. (2002). Clinical features and comorbidity of mood fluctuations in Parkinson's disease. *Journal of Neuropsychiatry and Clinical Neurosciences, 14*(4), 438−442.

Reijnders, J. S., Ehrt, U., Weber, W. E., Aarsland, D., & Leentjens, A. F. (2008). A systematic review of prevalence studies of depression in Parkinson's disease. *Movement Disorders: Official Journal of the Movement Disorder Society, 23*(2), 183−189. quiz 313.

Richard, I. H., McDermott, M. P., Kurlan, R., Lyness, J. M., Como, P. G., Pearson, N., et al. (2012). A randomized, double-blind, placebo-controlled trial of antidepressants in Parkinson disease. *Neurology, 78*(16), 1229−1236.

Rutten, S., Vriend, C., van der Werf, Y. D., Berendse, H. W., Weintraub, D., & van den Heuvel, O. A. (2017). The bidirectional longitudinal relationship between insomnia, depression and anxiety in patients with early-stage, medication-naive Parkinson's disease. *Parkinsonism & Related Disorders, 39*, 31−36.

Shafazand, S., Wallace, D. M., Arheart, K. L., Vargas, S., Luca, C. C., Moore, H., et al. (2017). Insomnia, sleep quality, and quality of life in mild to moderate Parkinson's disease. *Annals of the American Thoracic Society, 14*(3), 412−419.

Singareddy, R., & Uhde, T. W. (2009). Nocturnal sleep panic and depression: Relationship to subjective sleep in panic disorder. *Journal of Affective Disorders, 112*(1−3), 262−266.

Suzuki, K., Miyamoto, M., Miyamoto, T., Okuma, Y., Hattori, N., Kamei, S., et al. (2009). Correlation between depressive symptoms and nocturnal disturbances in Japanese patients with Parkinson's disease. *Parkinsonism & Related Disorders, 15*(1), 15−19.

Vazquez, A., Jimenez-Jimenez, F. J., Garcia-Ruiz, P., & Garcia-Urra, D. (1993). "Panic attacks" in Parkinson's disease. A long-term complication of levodopa therapy. *Acta Neurologica Scandinavica, 87*(1), 14−18.

Verbaan, D., van Rooden, S. M., Visser, M., Marinus, J., & van Hilten, J. J. (2008). Nighttime sleep problems and daytime sleepiness in Parkinson's disease. *Movement Disorders: Official Journal of the Movement Disorder Society, 23*(1), 35−41.

Yong, M. H., Fook-Chong, S., Pavanni, R., Lim, L. L., & Tan, E. K. (2011). Case control polysomnographic studies of sleep disorders in Parkinson's disease. *PLoS One, 6*(7), e22511.

Yu, S. Y., Sun, L., Liu, Z., Huang, X. Y., Zuo, L. J., Cao, C. J., et al. (2013). Sleep disorders in Parkinson's disease: Clinical features, iron metabolism and related mechanism. *PLoS One, 8*(12), e82924.

Nocturnal psychosis

Illustrative case

A 77-year-old man with Parkinson's disease (PD) and dementia presents to his neurologist accompanied by his wife. His motor symptoms are reasonably well controlled with levodopa 200 mg four times a day. Nonmotor issues include overactive bladder for which he has been on oxybutynin for years. He has mild dementia; he is more forgetful and sometimes gets confused and disoriented, particularly after he wakes up from daytime naps, and in the evenings. He is, however, still largely independent of activities of daily living. His wife is concerned, though, because there have been several incidents at night that are very concerning to her. On one occasion, he thought that he had heard intruders in the house; she woke up to find him on the phone with the police asking them to come and investigate. In another instance, she woke up to the sound of him yelling and hitting at something and when she turned the lights on, he was pounding a chair in their bedroom against the wall. He reported to her that he had thought that it was someone in their bedroom. After redirection and reassurance, he had acknowledged that this may all have been in his imagination. There were several similar episodes, and they had increased in frequency in recent months.

Overview

Definition

Psychosis is defined by the presence of symptoms suggestive of impaired awareness and understanding of reality. These symptoms include hallucinations and delusions. Hallucinations are abnormal perceptions without a physical stimulus, which can involve any sensory modality, and without retained insight. Delusions are false fixed beliefs that are maintained despite evidence of the contrary. Other criteria for diagnosis of psychosis in primary psychotic disorders (such as schizophrenia) include disorganized behavior (American Psychiatric Association, 2013).

In PD patients with psychosis, visual hallucinations are the most common manifestation. They are often well formed and often consist of people or animals

Disorders of Sleep and Wakefulness in Parkinson's Disease. https://doi.org/10.1016/B978-0-323-67374-7.00004-3

(Fenelon & Alves, 2010; Fenelon, Mahieux, Huon, & Ziegler, 2000; Fenelon, Soulas, Zenasni, & Cleret de Langavant, 2010; Ravina et al., 2007; Sanchez-Ramos, Ortoll, & Paulson, 1996). Auditory, olfactory, and tactile hallucinations occur in PD as well, though often in association with visual hallucinations and rarely in isolation (Fenelon et al., 2000; Inzelberg, Kipervasser, & Korczyn, 1998). Another type of hallucination in PD is presence phenomenon, whereby the patient experiences the presence of someone when no one is really there. Related is the passage phenomenon, which is marked by a vision of the transient passage of a person or animal. Passage and presence phenomena have been called "minor" hallucinations in some studies (Fenelon et al., 2000). Illusions also occur in PD, which are misperceptions of existing stimuli.

Diagnostic criteria for psychosis in PD have been put forth (Ravina et al., 2007). These require the presence of at least one psychotic symptom (illusions, false sense of presence, hallucinations, delusions) lasting for at least 1 month, unexplained by other conditions, along with a diagnosis of PD based on clinical criteria. According to these criteria, PD psychosis is further qualified by associated features of dementia, or whether there is a treatment-induced etiology.

In relation to sleep, psychosis in PD may have a preponderance for occurring during the evening ("sun-downing") and/or during the night (hereto forth called as "nocturnal psychosis"). Psychotic symptoms may be temporally related to daytime sleep as well (Arnulf et al., 2000), as further discussed later.

Epidemiology

Data on the epidemiology of psychosis in PD vary based on the definition used and the population sampled Fenelon and Alves (2010). Point prevalence in community-based samples of PD patients has ranged from 16% to 50%; rates of 50% have also been reported in clinic-based samples. As for lifetime prevalence rates, reports range from 25% to 60% (Aarsland, Larsen, Cummins, & Laake, 1999; Fenelon & Alves, 2010; Fenelon et al., 2000; Forsaa et al., 2010; Hely, Morris, Reid, & Trafficante, 2005; Pacchetti et al., 2005).

As for the prevalence of sleep-related psychosis, data are further limited. What data are available suggest that in patients with psychosis, nocturnal symptoms of psychosis are very common (Barnes, Connelly, Wiggs, Boubert, & Maravic, 2010; Pacchetti et al., 2005; Sanchez-Ramos et al., 1996; Whitehead, Davies, Playfer, & Turnbull, 2008). In a study of 289 outpatients with PD (Pacchetti et al., 2005), sleep and psychosis history were ascertained via interview and a questionnaire: 92 (32%) reported psychotic symptoms, with 86 (93%) of those reporting hallucinations. In turn, 62 (72%) of hallucinators reported nocturnal hallucinations. Regarding the timing of nocturnal hallucinations, in some patients, nocturnal hallucinations coincided with nocturnal awakenings (so-called hypnopompic hallucinations); whereas, in other patients they occurred during established nocturnal wakefulness. Interestingly, some patients also report hypnopompic hallucinations following awakening from daytime naps. Many patients report nocturnal hallucinations are more likely to occur in the dark and resolve when lights are turned on (Pacchetti et al., 2005).

Furthermore, data indicate that psychosis is more common in PD patients with sleep problems (Fenelon et al., 2000; Whitehead et al., 2008). In one study that recruited from a large population of PD patients presenting to one of two outpatient clinics in France, 216 PD patients were assessed (Fenelon et al., 2000). Prevalence of hallucinations was determined via interview, as was history of sleep disturbances. "Severe sleep disturbance" was marked by the presence of two or more of the following: difficulty falling asleep or more than one awakening from sleep; early morning awakening; nocturnal agitation; and vivid dreams. Mean disease duration was 9.5 years, and 20% had dementia. Moreover, 40% of the sample reported hallucinations in the preceding 3 months (Fenelon et al., 2000). Severe sleep disturbances occurred in 31.2% of those with visual hallucinations versus 18.6% of those without visual hallucinations, though this difference was not statistically significant.

Once hallucinations in PD occur, they are usually persistent (Goetz, Wuu, Curgian, & Leurgans, 2005), especially in patients with cognitive impairment and dementia. However, in some cases, they may improve or even resolve with adjustment of dopaminergic medications or other interventions.

Etiology and differential diagnosis

Several risk factors for PD psychosis have been identified, and these are similarly risk factors for nocturnal psychosis in PD (Table 4.1) (Baker et al., 2009; Fenelon & Alves, 2010; Fenelon et al., 2000; Forsaa et al., 2010; Lee & Weintraub, 2012; Ravina et al., 2007; Stowe et al., 2008).

Psychosis is more common in older PD patients and PD patients with longer disease duration (Fenelon & Alves, 2010; Fenelon et al., 2000; Ravina et al., 2007). Indeed, occurrence of hallucinations within 1 year of diagnosis may suggest an alternate diagnosis (namely, Dementia with Lewy Bodies) (Fenelon et al., 2000; Goetz, Vogel, Tanner, & Stebbins, 1998). Greater motor severity is also seen in patients with PD psychosis (Fenelon & Alves, 2010; Fenelon et al., 2000).

Accounting for confounding by disease severity and other factors, data indicate that treatment with dopaminergic medications is a risk factor for PD psychosis (Fenelon & Alves, 2010; Fenelon et al., 2000). Both dopamine agonists and levodopa can cause or exacerbate PD psychosis, though dopamine agonists are particularly likely to do so, especially in older patients. Two meta-analyses of data from randomized trials of dopamine agonists in early PD demonstrated a higher risk of hallucinations in PD patients treated with an agonist as compared to placebo, or levodopa (Baker et al., 2009; Stowe et al., 2008).

In a study that aimed to assess the prospective relationship between sleep problems and hallucinations in PD (Goetz et al., 2005), a group of 89 patients were recruited from an outpatient movement disorders clinic, based on their membership in one of five groups defined as follows: presence of sleep fragmentation, vivid

Table 4.1 Risk factors for PD psychosis.

Risk factor	Comment
Age	Older age is associated with psychosis in PD
Disease duration	Psychosis in PD typically occurs after several years' disease duration
Advanced disease	Psychosis in PD is associated with greater motor disease severity
Neuropsychiatric symptoms	Cognitive dysfunction/dementia and psychosis are often comorbid in PD. Cognitive dysfunction can also be seen as a risk factor for PD psychosis
	Depression is associated with increased risk of psychosis in PD
Sleep disorders	REM sleep behavior disorder is strongly associated with increased risk of PD psychosis
Visual acuity	Reduced visual acuity is associated with higher probability of visual hallucinations in PD
Medications	
Anticholinergics	Several medications used to treat nonmotor symptoms in PD have anticholinergic properties. Consideration for cumulative "anticholinergic burden" is essential in such instances
Amantadine	Amantadine likely is associated with psychosis due to anticholinergic effects but may also predispose to psychosis related to dopaminergic or other effects
	Amantadine-induced psychosis is more likely in older adults and in those with kidney dysfunction
	Importantly, abrupt amantadine withdrawal can also be associated with confusion/hallucinations
Dopaminergic medications	Dopamine agonists > levodopa
Other	Analgesics, antihistamines

dreams/nightmares, hallucinations with retained insight, hallucinations without retained insight, and normal sleep without hallucinations. Symptoms of sleep were assessed by structured interview and the Pittsburgh Sleep Quality Index (PSQI). Symptoms of psychosis were assessed by the Rush PD Behavioral Interview. 73 had an at least 18-month follow-up assessment and 49 were assessed at 72 months from baseline. Over 6 years, the prevalence of hallucinators increased from 33% at baseline to 55% at 72 months, and 42% had severe hallucinations on at least one follow-up interview. Although sleep problems did not predict new-onset hallucinations, presence of vivid dreams/nightmares at a given visit was strongly associated with risk of hallucinations at the same visit (Goetz et al., 2005).

Several studies have also demonstrated increased prevalence of REM sleep behavior disorder (RBD) in individuals with hallucinations, and increased risk of hallucinations in PD patients with RBD, across all disease stages (Ffytche et al., 2017; Forsaa et al., 2010; Lenka, Hegde, Jhunjhunwala, & Pal, 2016; Pacchetti et al., 2005). A direct pathophysiologic relationship between hallucinations and abnormal sleep, and specifically in relation to REM sleep, has been posited in PD. Based on the observed close relationship between vivid dreams/nightmares in PD and risk of hallucinations, it has been hypothesized that psychosis in PD may result from abnormal REM sleep. A strong temporal association between occurrence of REM periods and occurrence of hallucinations during presumed wakefulness has been reported. Indeed, in a study examining daytime sleepiness via multiple sleep latency test in 10 PD, daytime sleepiness with REM periods during daytime sleep episodes was associated with hallucinations (Arnulf et al., 2000). Further supporting this possibility is that PD patients who hallucinate are more likely to have other abnormal REM manifestations including increased muscle tone in REM. Patients with hallucinations and vivid dreams often report having difficulty distinguishing between whether they are awake or asleep when they "see things" at night, and it is possible that indeed they are in an intermediate state between wakefulness and REM sleep, "where dream content was still vivid although mixed with reality" (Arnulf et al., 2000).

In cross-sectional studies, comorbidity of PD psychosis with several nonmotor features including depression and anxiety have been described (Fenelon et al., 2000), and when these are all concurrently present, these may individually or synergistically exacerbate sleep in PD (see Chapter 3 for more on the relationship of depression and anxiety on sleep in PD). Daytime hypersomnolence is also greater in PD patients with psychosis compared to those without (Barnes et al., 2010; Fenelon et al., 2000; Pacchetti et al., 2005) (see Chapter 12 for more on excessive daytime sleepiness in PD). Daytime hallucinations in PD may occur during awakenings from daytime naps (Pacchetti et al., 2005).

Cognitive dysfunction and especially dementia are also commonly comorbid with PD psychosis (Fenelon et al., 2000). Moreover, 70% of PD patients with dementia report hallucinations. Beyond being a common comorbidity, cognitive dysfunction/dementia serve as a risk factor for psychosis in PD as well, given that cognitive dysfunction may alter awareness and perceptions of environmental stimuli (Arnulf et al., 2000). When comorbid, cognitive dysfunction and psychosis can impact sleep in PD by leading to sleep onset and maintenance insomnia, nocturnal agitation, and are a risk factor for nocturnal wandering.

Hallucinations in the absence of dementia are less common, but certainly still occur, in about 20%−30% of PD patients without cognitive dysfunction (Barrett et al., 2017; Lee & Weintraub, 2012). In a cross-sectional study of 192 nondemented PD patients, psychotic symptoms were ascertained via a detailed interview and rater-administered Parkinson's Psychosis Rating Scale. Psychosis was present in 21.5% of the sample. Of note, over half of the cohort was being treated with dopamine agonists, with no difference between the hallucinators and nonhallucinators. Patients with comorbid depression and daytime sleepiness had five times the odds of having psychotic symptoms (Lee & Weintraub, 2012). In contrast, another study assessing for psychosis in PD patients with normal cognition found dopamine agonist use to be a risk factor for psychotic symptoms. This study also replicated the finding that in PD patients without cognitive impairment, RBD is an independent predictor of hallucinations (Barrett et al., 2017). In early, untreated PD, visual hallucinations are associated with amyloid pathology (as ascertained by CSF analysis) (Pereira et al., 2014). Several lines of evidence indeed indicate that RBD and/or hallucinations in PD patients without cognitive impairment are harbingers of dementia, or at a minimum suggest an increased risk for it (Anang et al., 2014; Chahine et al., 2016; de la Riva Smith, Xie, & Weintraub, 2014; Ffytche et al., 2017).

One study found that hallucinations were more likely in PD patients whose RBD preceded their motor manifestations (as opposed to RBD starting after PD was diagnosed) (Pacchetti et al., 2005). This lends support to another hypothesis relating to the relationship between RBD and more severe neuropsychiatric manifestations, namely that RBD reflects more severe and/or more widespread neurodegeneration that in turn manifests with hallucinations, cognitive impairment, and other features. Indeed, volumetric MRI studies greater atrophy in the hippocampus and parahippocampus in PD patients with RBD and hallucinations (Lenka et al., 2016). Abnormalities in cholinergic transmission may also be implicated (Hilker et al., 2005; Lenka et al., 2016). See Chapter 6 for more on RBD as a prodromal feature to PD, and Chapter 5 for more on RBD in PD.

Consequences and complications

As described earlier, several studies have indicated that PD patients with psychosis have more nocturnal sleep problems and daytime sleepiness compared to those without (Barnes et al., 2010; Pappert, Goetz, Niederman, Raman, & Leurgans, 1999). PD patients with psychosis have abnormalities in nocturnal and daytime activity levels, a measure of circadian rhythm. In one study, measurement of so-called "rest-activity levels" (RAR) was achieved with actigraphy in 50 PD patients and 29 healthy controls, and compared in PD patients with versus without hallucination (Whitehead et al., 2008). History of hallucinations was ascertained with semistructured interview. Hallucinators had greater nocturnal activity levels, a measure of disturbed nocturnal sleep. Hallucinators also had less predictable activity patterns during the day. In another study, a history of visual hallucinations was ascertained via questionnaire and used to identify 17 PD patients with psychosis and 17 PD patients without (Barnes et al., 2010). Twenty non-PD controls were also included. Wrist actigraphy was performed for 5 days; sleep history and symptoms were also ascertained via sleep diary and PSQI. Hallucinators had more daytime sleepiness, especially unexpected sleepiness (Barnes et al., 2010). Hallucinators also had less sleep efficiency, more awake time at night, and more periods of wakefulness after sleep onset as compared to PD patients without hallucinations and controls.

Nocturnal psychosis in PD can lead to fear, anxiety, and worry in patients (Pacchetti et al., 2005). PD psychosis, including, and perhaps especially sleep-related psychosis, leads to significant caregiver burden (Fenelon & Alves, 2010; Ravina et al., 2007). Unfortunately, there can be extreme manifestations of nocturnal psychosis in PD, including combativeness (Bliwise et al., 1995). This may be more likely in PD patients with cognitive dysfunction.

Management

The management of nocturnal psychosis in PD requires a multifaceted approach (Table 4.2).

Where there are comorbid sleep disorders such as RBD and or sleep apnea, their separate treatment is needed as well, as discussed in their respective chapters. As discussed, it has been hypothesized that at least in some instances nocturnal psychosis is related to, if not directly results from, abnormal REM phenomena related to RBD. Thus, controlling RBD symptoms may help reduce nocturnal psychosis. Treating sleep apnea may reduce sleep fragmentation and nighttime awakenings which in turn has the potential to reduce nocturnal psychosis.

Treatment of other comorbidities such as anxiety and depression is indicated. In addition, for patients with cognitive dysfunction, use of an acetylcholine esterase

Table 4.2 Management of nocturnal psychosis in PD.

Therapeutic strategy	Comment
Treatment of comorbid sleep disorders	Treatment of comorbid sleep disorders such as REM sleep behavior disorder could help to reduce nocturnal psychosis. Treating sleep apnea may reduce sleep fragmentation and nighttime awakenings
Treatment of comorbid neuropsychiatric symptoms	Treatment of comorbid depression, anxiety, and cognitive dysfunction may improve nocturnal psychosis symptoms in PD
Optimizing the environment	Simplifying the bedroom, removing any unnecessary furniture and obstacles, is ideal. Ensuring quick access to full-bedroom illumination may be beneficial as well. Motion-sensitive lights could be of use in this regard
Optimizing dopaminergic medications	Anticholinergic burden must be minimized and eliminated where possible. In patients with nocturnal psychosis, reduction of dopamine agonists and their cessation may be necessary Reducing levodopa dose may eventually be required; balance between mitigating psychosis and controlling motor symptoms will have to be achieved on a case-by-case basis
Use of antipsychotics	Judicious use of antipsychotics may be required in instances where other measures are not sufficient and where significant distress or safety concerns, on the part of the patient or caregivers, arise. Use of antipsychotics with low potency of antagonism at dopamine receptors, such as clozapine and quetiapine, is necessary to avoid exacerbating parkinsonism. Pimavanserin may be of utility for nocturnal psychosis in PD as well

inhibitor would be appropriate and could help to reduce some of the behavioral symptoms (Pagano et al., 2015), as well as caregiver burden.

A few studies and anecdotal data indicate that nocturnal PD psychosis is often precipitated or at least exacerbated by the bedroom environment. Specifically, patients often report misperceiving shadows from various objects in the bedroom including hung clothes or bedroom furniture. Patients also report that hallucinations typically occur in dark or low-light conditions and sometimes are completely resolved just by turning the lights on (Pacchetti et al., 2005) (suggesting that illusions factor into nocturnal PD psychosis). Therefore, where possible, simplifying the bedroom environment, and ensuring that lights can be quickly turned on to illuminate the room quickly in its entirety may help to mitigate nocturnal illusions and even hallucinations.

Although psychosis in PD may be independent of PD treatment, as mentioned earlier, dopaminergic medications, and especially dopamine agonists, may induce psychosis and/or exacerbate it. Therefore, another critical step in management of PD psychosis is to stop dopamine agonists, and reduce levodopa where possible (Fenelon & Alves, 2010; Ravina et al., 2007). For patients with nocturnal psychosis, sometimes lowering the evening dose of dopaminergic medications may help. Certainly, a balance between optimizing treatment of motor symptoms and mitigating any side effects of dopaminergic medications is always needed in PD.

When nocturnal psychosis is disruptive to the patients' and caregivers sleep, leads to significant distress for either, and/or puts them at risk for compromised safety, if the earlier interventions are not sufficient, pharmacotherapy specifically targeting psychosis may be indicated. Use of antipsychotics in PD requires careful consideration, as most antipsychotics block dopamine, which can exacerbate parkinsonism. Use of antipsychotics has been associated with increased morbidity and increased risk of mortality in PD (Weintraub et al., 2016, 2017). Although this could reflect more severe disease burden rather than a direct effect of antipsychotics, there is nevertheless a "black box" warning for increased risk of mortality for antipsychotic use in older adults that must be considered. Where necessary, use of antipsychotics with the least potency at dopamine receptors is indicated from that perspective. Relatively good level of evidence supports the efficacy and relative safety of clozapine for treatment of psychosis in PD, as appraised by the Movement Disorders Society evidence-based medicine review on treatments for nonmotor symptoms of PD (Seppi et al., 2019). Unfortunately, clozapine carries with it a risk of neutropenia, which is rare but can be severe and even life threatening. Therefore, monitoring with up to weekly complete blood count is necessary in the initial period of clozapine treatment, making it a less attractive therapeutic option for some patients and physicians. Quetiapine is another antipsychotic with relatively low dopamine blocking action. There are no high-quality randomized controlled trials to support its efficacy in PD but it is nevertheless considered possibly useful for treatment of psychosis in PD based on its mechanism of action (which is similar to clozapine) (Seppi et al., 2019) and anecdotal evidence.

A relatively newer addition to the armamentarium for treatment of PD psychosis is pimavanserin, an inverse agonist at the 5HT2A serotonin receptor. A post hoc analysis pooled data from two randomized, double-blind controlled studies of PD psychosis, one of which has been published by Cummings et al. (2013). This post hoc analysis included data from 187 PD patients who received pimavanserin and 187 PD patients who received placebo (Patel et al., 2018). Significant improvements in nighttime sleep scores were observed among patients who had reported impaired nighttime sleep and daytime sleepiness.

Illustrative case in context

In the case presented, the patient is a 77-year-old man with Parkinson's disease dementia and nocturnal psychosis. He is having what sounds like nocturnal auditory and visual hallucinations that are very disruptive and could put both him and his wife at risk of harm. Initial treatment would include evaluation by an urologist to see if the oxybutynin could be replaced with a medication with less anticholinergic properties. Consideration for donepezil may be appropriate in his case, as it could improve or at least stabilize his daytime cognitive dysfunction as well as the behavioral problems. In addition, it may be appropriate to lower his levodopa; to minimize a significant negative impact on his motor function, perhaps just the amount he takes for his fourth dose may be reduced, as he is more likely to have psychosis symptoms in the evening and night. Modification of his bedroom environment to reduce any unnecessary furniture and other stimuli that may be misperceived would be helpful. Finally, if these interventions fail, he may benefit from pharmacotherapy. In this case, pimavanserin may be of use, or quetiapine. If those medications do not help, the potential risks and inconvenience of clozapine may be out weighed by its potential benefit.

References

Aarsland, D., Larsen, J. P., Cummins, J. L., & Laake, K. (1999). Prevalence and clinical correlates of psychotic symptoms in Parkinson disease: A community-based study. *Archives of Neurology, 56*(5), 595−601.

American Psychiatric Association. (2013). *Diagnostic and statistical manual of mental disorders* (5th ed.). Arlington, VA: American Psychiatric Publishing.

Anang, J. B., Gagnon, J. F., Bertrand, J. A., Romenets, S. R., Latreille, V., Panisset, M., et al. (2014). Predictors of dementia in Parkinson disease: A prospective cohort study. *Neurology, 83*(14), 1253−1260.

Arnulf, I., Bonnet, A. M., Damier, P., Bejjani, B. P., Seilhean, D., Derenne, J. P., et al. (2000). Hallucinations, REM sleep, and Parkinson's disease: A medical hypothesis. *Neurology, 55*(2), 281−288.

Baker, W. L., Silver, D., White, C. M., Kluger, J., Aberle, J., Patel, A. A., et al. (2009). Dopamine agonists in the treatment of early Parkinson's disease: A meta-analysis. *Parkinsonism & Related Disorders, 15*(4), 287−294.

Barnes, J., Connelly, V., Wiggs, L., Boubert, L., & Maravic, K. (2010). Sleep patterns in Parkinson's disease patients with visual hallucinations. *The International Journal of Neuroscience, 120*(8), 564–569.

Barrett, M. J., Smolkin, M. E., Flanigan, J. L., Shah, B. B., Harrison, M. B., & Sperling, S. A. (2017). Characteristics, correlates, and assessment of psychosis in Parkinson disease without dementia. *Parkinsonism & Related Disorders, 43*, 56–60.

Bliwise, D. L., Watts, R. L., Watts, N., Rye, D. B., Irbe, D., & Hughes, M. (1995). Disruptive nocturnal behavior in Parkinson's disease and Alzheimer's disease. *Journal of Geriatric Psychiatry and Neurology, 8*(2), 107–110.

Chahine, L. M., Xie, S. X., Simuni, T., Tran, B., Postuma, R., Amara, A., et al. (2016). Longitudinal changes in cognition in early Parkinson's disease patients with REM sleep behavior disorder. *Parkinsonism & Related Disorders*.

Cummings, J., Isaacson, S., Mills, R., Williams, H., Chi-Burris, K., Corbett, A., et al. (2013). Pimavanserin for patients with Parkinson's disease psychosis: A randomised, placebo-controlled phase 3 trial. *Lancet*.

Fenelon, G., & Alves, G. (2010). Epidemiology of psychosis in Parkinson's disease. *Journal of the Neurological Sciences, 289*(1–2), 12–17.

Fenelon, G., Mahieux, F., Huon, R., & Ziegler, M. (2000). Hallucinations in Parkinson's disease: Prevalence, phenomenology and risk factors. *Brain: Journal of Neurology, 123*(Pt 4), 733–745.

Fenelon, G., Soulas, T., Zenasni, F., & Cleret de Langavant, L. (2010). The changing face of Parkinson's disease-associated psychosis: A cross-sectional study based on the new NINDS-NIMH criteria. *Movement Disorders: Official Journal of the Movement Disorder Society, 25*(6), 763–766.

Ffytche, D. H., Pereira, J. B., Ballard, C., Chaudhuri, K. R., Weintraub, D., & Aarsland, D. (2017). Risk factors for early psychosis in PD: Insights from the Parkinson's progression markers initiative. *Journal of Neurology, Neurosurgery & Psychiatry, 88*(4), 325–331.

Forsaa, E. B., Larsen, J. P., Wentzel-Larsen, T., Goetz, C. G., Stebbins, G. T., Aarsland, D., et al. (2010). A 12-year population-based study of psychosis in Parkinson disease. *Archives of Neurology, 67*(8), 996–1001.

Goetz, C. G., Vogel, C., Tanner, C. M., & Stebbins, G. T. (1998). Early dopaminergic drug-induced hallucinations in parkinsonian patients. *Neurology, 51*(3), 811–814.

Goetz, C. G., Wuu, J., Curgian, L. M., & Leurgans, S. (2005). Hallucinations and sleep disorders in PD: Six-year prospective longitudinal study. *Neurology, 64*(1), 81–86.

Hely, M. A., Morris, J. G., Reid, W. G., & Trafficante, R. (2005). Sydney multicenter study of Parkinson's disease: Non-l-dopa-responsive problems dominate at 15 years. *Movement Disorders: Official Journal of the Movement Disorder Society, 20*(2), 190–199.

Hilker, R., Thomas, A. V., Klein, J. C., Weisenbach, S., Kalbe, E., Burghaus, L., et al. (2005). Dementia in Parkinson disease: Functional imaging of cholinergic and dopaminergic pathways. *Neurology, 65*(11), 1716–1722.

Inzelberg, R., Kipervasser, S., & Korczyn, A. D. (1998). Auditory hallucinations in Parkinson's disease. *Journal of Neurology, Neurosurgery & Psychiatry, 64*(4), 533–535.

Lee, A. H., & Weintraub, D. (2012). Psychosis in Parkinson's disease without dementia: Common and comorbid with other non-motor symptoms. *Movement Disorders: Official Journal of the Movement Disorder Society, 27*(7), 858–863.

Lenka, A., Hegde, S., Jhunjhunwala, K. R., & Pal, P. K. (2016). Interactions of visual hallucinations, rapid eye movement sleep behavior disorder and cognitive impairment in Parkinson's disease: A review. *Parkinsonism & Related Disorders, 22*, 1–8.

Pacchetti, C., Manni, R., Zangaglia, R., Mancini, F., Marchioni, E., Tassorelli, C., et al. (2005). Relationship between hallucinations, delusions, and rapid eye movement sleep behavior disorder in Parkinson's disease. *Movement Disorders: Official Journal of the Movement Disorder Society, 20*(11), 1439−1448.

Pagano, G., Rengo, G., Pasqualetti, G., Femminella, G. D., Monzani, F., Ferrara, N., et al. (2015). Cholinesterase inhibitors for Parkinson's disease: A systematic review and meta-analysis. *Journal of Neurology, Neurosurgery & Psychiatry, 86*(7), 767−773.

Pappert, E. J., Goetz, C. G., Niederman, F. G., Raman, R., & Leurgans, S. (1999). Hallucinations, sleep fragmentation, and altered dream phenomena in Parkinson's disease. *Movement Disorders: Official Journal of the Movement Disorder Society, 14*(1), 117−121.

Patel, N., LeWitt, P., Neikrug, A. B., Kesslak, P., Coate, B., & Ancoli-Israel, S. (2018). Nighttime sleep and daytime sleepiness improved with pimavanserin during treatment of Parkinson's disease psychosis. *Clinical Neuropharmacology, 41*(6), 210−215.

Pereira, J. B., Svenningsson, P., Weintraub, D., Bronnick, K., Lebedev, A., Westman, E., et al. (2014). Initial cognitive decline is associated with cortical thinning in early Parkinson disease. *Neurology, 82*(22), 2017−2025.

Ravina, B., Marder, K., Fernandez, H. H., Friedman, J. H., McDonald, W., Murphy, D., et al. (2007). Diagnostic criteria for psychosis in Parkinson's disease: Report of an NINDS, NIMH work group. *Movement Disorders: Official Journal of the Movement Disorder Society, 22*(8), 1061−1068.

de la Riva, P., Smith, K., Xie, S. X., & Weintraub, D. (2014). Course of psychiatric symptoms and global cognition in early Parkinson disease. *Neurology, 83*(12), 1096−1103.

Sanchez-Ramos, J. R., Ortoll, R., & Paulson, G. W. (1996). Visual hallucinations associated with Parkinson disease. *Archives of Neurology, 53*(12), 1265−1268.

Seppi, K., Ray Chaudhuri, K., Coelho, M., Fox, S. H., Katzenschlager, R., Perez Lloret, S., et al. (2019). Update on treatments for nonmotor symptoms of Parkinson's disease-an evidence-based medicine review. *Movement Disorders: Official Journal of the Movement Disorder Society, 34*(2), 180−198.

Stowe, R. L., Ives, N. J., Clarke, C., van Hilten, J., Ferreira, J., Hawker, R. J., et al. (2008). Dopamine agonist therapy in early Parkinson's disease. *The Cochrane Database of Systematic Reviews*, (2), CD006564.

Weintraub, D., Chiang, C., Kim, H. M., Wilkinson, J., Marras, C., Stanislawski, B., et al. (2016). Association of antipsychotic use with mortality risk in patients with Parkinson disease. *JAMA Neurology, 73*(5), 535−541.

Weintraub, D., Chiang, C., Kim, H. M., Wilkinson, J., Marras, C., Stanislawski, B., et al. (2017). Antipsychotic use and physical morbidity in Parkinson disease. *The American Journal of Geriatric Psychiatry: Official Journal of the American Association for Geriatric Psychiatry*.

Whitehead, D. L., Davies, A. D., Playfer, J. R., & Turnbull, C. J. (2008). Circadian rest-activity rhythm is altered in Parkinson's disease patients with hallucinations. *Movement Disorders: Official Journal of the Movement Disorder Society, 23*(8), 1137−1145.

REM sleep behavior disorder in Parkinson's disease

Illustrative case

A 69-year-old man with Parkinson's disease (PD) diagnosed 2 years earlier presents to the emergency department with bruising and swelling around his eye after falling out of bed. He reports that he was dreaming of chasing a burglar and woke up to find himself on the floor. His wife reports that for years, he has talked in his sleep and occasionally thrashed out or kicked; he has frequent recall of dreams in which he is fighting someone. Of note, he recently was started on mirtazapine at bedtime for anxiety and depression.

Overview

Definition

REM sleep behavior disorder (RBD) is a rapid eye movement (REM) parasomnia that manifest clinically with dream enactment behavior and electrophysiologically, on surface electromyography (EMG), with REM without atonia (RWA) (American Academy of Sleep Medicine, 2014). Dream enactment varies but often manifests with vocalizations and movements that often appear purposeful. Dream content in RBD is often violent, and patients therefore often manifest fighting movements (punching, kicking) (Bjornara, Dietrichs, & Toft, 2013). Of note, during dream enactments, patients may execute movements and have louder vocalizations than are seen during wakefulness (De Cock et al., 2007).

As for the RWA, as discussed in Chapter 6, REM sleep is marked by loss of activity in most muscle groups. There is atonia, essentially paralysis, of most muscle groups, with notable exceptions including the diaphragm and extraocular movements. A loss of that atonia, RWA, is the electrophysiologic signature of RBD. RWA may manifest with either tonic increases in EMG activity or several phasic increases (Montplaisir et al., 2010). The definition of what constitutes RWA on a quantitative versus qualitative basis is a matter of debate and ongoing research (Ferri, Fulda, Cosentino, Pizza, & Plazzi, 2012; Kempfner, Sorensen, Zoetmulder, Jennum, & Sorensen, 2010; McCarter, St Louis, Duwell et al., 2014; Sixel-Doring,

Schweitzer, Mollenhauer, & Trenkwalder, 2011). Normative data on the degree of surface EMG activity seen in different age groups and in men versus women have been used to determine the degree of muscle activity in REM that is consistent with RBD (Frauscher et al., 2012).

A diagnosis of RBD is made based on the presence of RWA combined with a history of dream enactment behavior (not explained by other disorders) and/or video-polysomnographic evidence of dream enactment (American Academy of Sleep Medicine, 2018). A diagnosis of possible RBD (pRBD) may be made based on questionnaire (Chahine et al., 2013; Frauscher et al., 2014; Nomura, Inoue, Kagimura, Uemura, & Nakashima, 2011; Postuma, Arnulf et al., 2012; Shen et al., 2014; Stiasny-Kolster et al., 2007, 2015). These questionnaires were largely developed to detect RBD in patients without diagnosed neurodegenerative parkinsonisms, and available questionnaires may lack sensitivity and specificity for RBD in PD (Chahine et al., 2013; Li, Li, Su, & Chen, 2017; Stefani et al., 2016), especially in early PD (Halsband, Zapf, Sixel-Doring, Trenkwalder, & Mollenhauer, 2018). Many patients with pRBD (questionnaire-based RBD) do not have RWA (Bolitho et al., 2014). Therefore, interpretation of findings based on questionnaire-based diagnosis of RBD (without polysomnographic confirmation) in PD requires caution. Input of a bed partner/roommate does improve specificity and sensitivity of questionnaire-based diagnosis (Boeve et al., 2011; Chahine et al., 2013). As for other objective measures of RBD, actigraphy, a measure of nocturnal mobility, shows a good specificity but a low sensitivity for diagnosis (Louter, Arends, Bloem, & Overeem, 2014).

RBD as a manifestation of prodromal PD is discussed in Chapter 6.

Epidemiology

RBD is common in PD. In PD cohorts evaluated at tertiary care centers, the prevalence of RBD (with polysomnographic confirmation of RWA) is 39%—46% (Neikrug et al., 2013; Sixel-Doring, Trautmann, Mollenhauer, & Trenkwalder, 2011). In early PD cohorts prevalence is lower, with pRBD identified (with questionnaire) in 20%—25% (Chahine et al., 2016; Liu et al., 2019) and polysomnographically confirmed RBD occurring in approximately one-third of patients (Plomhause et al., 2013). If the definition of RBD is liberalized to only require purposeful motor behaviors and/or vocalizations in REM sleep (irrespective of RWA), these occur in about 50% of early PD patients (Sixel-Doring, Trautmann, Mollenhauer, & Trenkwalder, 2014).

Studies indicate that RBD is more common in male PD patients compared to females (Zhu, Xie, Hu, & Wang, 2017); of note, RBD may be underdiagnosed in females with PD (Mahale, Yadav, & Pal, 2016). In addition, the clinical manifestations may be different. For example, more violent dream content is reported in males versus females (Bjornara et al., 2013). RBD in PD is associated with longer disease duration (Gong et al., 2014; Sixel-Doring, Trautmann et al., 2011) but as mentioned it occurs in early PD (Pagano et al., 2018) and in prodromal phases as well, as discussed in Chapter 6.

Regarding the evolution of RBD in PD over time, what data are available indicate that once RBD begins, symptoms persist in most patients. A study ascertained pRBD, using the REM sleep behavior disorder questionnaire (Stiasny-Kolster et al., 2007), in 96 participants with PD at baseline and after 3 years of follow-up (Bjornara, Dietrichs, & Toft, 2015). The prevalence of pRBD increased from 39% of the cohort at baseline to 49% at year 3. Among those who had pRBD at baseline, 75% also had it at follow-up. Incident pRBD occurred in 17%.

Etiology and differential diagnosis

As detailed further later, PD patients with RBD have more severe manifestations than those without. This has been interpreted as reflecting more severe underlying neurodegeneration in PD with RBD compared to those without. Supporting this are the findings of reduced dopamine transporter binding on PET-CT (Chung, Lee, Lee, Lee, & Sohn, 2017) as well as greater cholinergic denervation (Kotagal et al., 2012) in PD patients with RBD or pRBD compared to those without. Volumetric MRI studies have found reduced thalamic (Salsone et al., 2014) and putamen (Kamps et al., 2018) volumes. A study of 69 PD patients with pRBD compared to 238 without confirmed lower volumes in the thalamus and putamen and demonstrated additional areas with reduced volumes in the pRBD group in the pontomesencephalic tegmentum, medullary reticular formation, and hypothalamus. These findings are of note considering the neuroanatomic regions implicated in RWA and dream enactment (see further later).

Other objective measures further support this. During wakefulness, PD patients with RBD have greater EEG slowing (Gagnon et al., 2004). In addition, there is a higher prevalence of a specific risk variant, rs3756063, in PD patients with pRBD compared to those without in the SNCA gene (the gene that codes for α-synuclein, a protein implicated in PD pathophysiology) (Bjornara, Pihlstrom, Dietrichs, & Toft, 2018). This raises the possibility that underlying genotype may increase susceptibility to more severe disease manifestations that include RBD.

Another study examined biomarker differences and progression in recently diagnosed PD patients with RBD compared to those without (Pagano et al., 2018). 412 PD patients were screened for RBD with the REM sleep behavior disorder questionnaire (RBDSQ) (Stiasny-Kolster et al., 2007), and 38% had pRBD using a liberal cutoff for this scale. PD patients with pRBD had lower (worse) CSF amyloid-β_{1-42}, and CSF amyloid-β_{1-42} levels correlated with RBDSQ score.

The pathophysiology of RBD is complex and not fully elucidated. Dysfunction of several brainstem nuclei, including the glutamatergic peri-locus coeruleus, has been implicated in RWA (Boeve et al., 2007; Garcia-Lorenzo et al., 2013; Kim et al., 2014). As for dream enactment, this likely requires involvement of more rostral locomotor centers. A resting state functional MRI study in 18 PD patients with RBD compared to 16 patients without revealed reduced spontaneous activity in primary motor cortex and premotor cortex in those with RBD (D. Li et al., 2017). A small study was able to perform "ictal" SPECT during an episodes of dream enactment in three patients with RBD, one of which had PD. Activation in the "bilateral premotor areas, the interhemispheric cleft, the periaqueductal area, the dorsal and ventral pons and the anterior lobe of the cerebellum" was seen. This finding is in contrast to activation patterns seen during movement in wakefulness, and suggest that the pathways that mediate dream enactment episodes during sleep bypass the basal ganglia (Mayer, Bitterlich, Kuwert, Ritt, & Stefan, 2015).

When approaching the differential diagnosis of complex motor behaviors during sleep in PD, RBD accounts for the largest proportion of them (Manni, Terzaghi, Repetto, Zangaglia, and Pacchetti, 2010). The differential diagnosis does include obstructive sleep apnea; apnea-related arousals can mimic RBD (Iranzo & Santamaria, 2005). See Chapter 8 for more on obstructive sleep apnea in PD. Another differential diagnosis in PD is periodic limb movements, which when large amplitude may be perceived by the patient or bed partner as purposeful kicking movements (Gaig, 2017). See Chapter 6 for more information on the differential diagnosis of RBD.

Consequences and complications

As mentioned, PD patients with RBD have more severe PD manifestations (Table 5.1). RBD in PD is associated with reduced QOL (Gong et al., 2014; Rolinski et al., 2014).

PD patients with RBD have more severe motor manifestations (Nomura, Kishi, & Nakashima, 2017; Sixel-Doring, Trautmann et al., 2011) and may be more likely

Table 5.1 Clinical features of PD patients with RBD compared to those without.

Category	Manifestation
Motor	More advanced Hoehn andand Yahr stage
	Higher motor score
	More axial involvement/less tremor
	Greater rate of decline in motor function
	More freezing of gait
	Higher requirements for dopaminergic medications
	More motor fluctuations
Neuropsychiatric	Higher risk of cognitive dysfunction and dementia
	Greater rate of decline in cognitive function
	Higher prevalence and greater risk of depression, anxiety, apathy, and psychosis
	Greater risk of impulse control disorders
Disorders of sleep and wakefulness	Daytime sleepiness
Autonomic	Higher prevalence of orthostatic hypotension, constipation, and erectile dysfunction

to have axial involvement (Gong et al., 2014). Rate of decline in PD patients with RBD may be greater as compared to those without (Bugalho & Viana-Baptista, 2013; Duarte Folle, Paul, Bronstein, Keener, & Ritz, 2019; Sommerauer et al., 2014). Along these lines, PD patients with RBD may be more likely to have the subtype of PD that is marked by less tremor and more postural instability and gait abnormalities (Kumru, Santamaria, Tolosa, & Iranzo, 2007; Postuma, Gagnon, Vendette, Charland, & Montplaisir, 2008a, 2008b) and symmetry of disease (Romenets et al., 2012). In turn, they may be more likely to have falls (Postuma et al., 2008a; Sixel-Doring, Trautmann et al., 2011) and freezing of gait (Gong et al., 2014; Romenets et al., 2012). As for the response of PD patients with RBD compared to those without to PD medications, some studies indicate less responsiveness to PD medications (Postuma et al., 2008b) and/or a requirement for higher dopaminergic medication doses (Gong et al., 2014; Sixel-Doring, Trautmann et al., 2011; Sixel-Doring, Trautmann, Mollenhauer, & Trenkwalder, 2012) though findings are not consistent in the literature (Aygun, Turkel, Onar, & Sunter, 2014; Benninger et al., 2010; Rolinski et al., 2014). Related to that, some data indicate that the risk of impulse control disorders, a consequence of exposure to dopaminergic therapy, is higher in PD patients with RBD compared to those without (Bellosta Diago, Lopez Del Val, Santos Lasaosa, Lopez Garcia, & Viloria Alebesque, 2017). PD patients with RBD may be more likely to have motor fluctuations (Sixel-Doring, Trautmann et al., 2011) and develop dyskinesias (Gong et al., 2014). Importantly, PD patients with pRBD may have worse outcomes following DBS compared to those without (Zibetti et al., 2010).

One study of 136 patients with PD that assessed for RBD via interview and polysomnography found RBD in 47 patients (Nomura et al., 2017). They compared the nine patients whose RBD preceded the diagnosis of PD to the 37 whose RBD emerged after the diagnosis of PD and found the latter group were at higher risk of cognitive impairment in spite of similar motor severity. Although recall bias may influence the results, they do indicate that it is possible that emergence of RBD after PD disease onset may have different consequences from occurrence of RBD first, perhaps reflecting differences in the spatial progression of pathology (Parkkinen, Pirttila, & Alafuzoff, 2008).

Several nonmotor features are also more common in PD patients with RBD compared to those without. Notably, cognitive impairment is more prevalent (Gagnon et al., 2009; Gaudreault et al., 2013; Jozwiak et al., 2017; Marques et al., 2010; Pagano et al., 2018; Plomhause et al., 2014; Sinforiani et al., 2006; Terzaghi et al., 2013; Vendette et al., 2007), as is the rate of cognitive decline and risk of dementia (Anang et al., 2014; Duarte Folle et al., 2019; Jozwiak et al., 2017; Postuma, Bertrand et al., 2012; Sinforiani et al., 2008). In addition, PD patients with pRBD and RBD are more likely to experience depression (Bargiotas et al., 2019; Liu et al., 2017; Neikrug et al., 2013; Pagano et al., 2018; Romenets et al., 2012), fatigue (Neikrug et al., 2013), apathy (Bargiotas et al., 2019), and psychosis (Forsaa et al., 2010; Pacchetti et al., 2005; Sinforiani et al., 2008; Sixel-Doring, Trautmann et al.,

2011). See Chapter 3 for more on depression in PD and Chapter 4 for more on nocturnal psychosis in PD.

Autonomic manifestations are also more severe in PD patients with RBD compared to those without. There is greater prevalence of orthostatic hypotension (Kim et al., 2016; Postuma, Gagnon, Pelletier, & Montplaisir, 2013; Postuma et al., 2008a; Romenets et al., 2012), reduced heart rate variability (Postuma, Lanfranchi, Blais, Gagnon, & Montplaisir, 2010; Postuma et al., 2011), constipation (Liu et al., 2017; Nihei et al., 2012; Postuma et al., 2013; Romenets et al., 2012), and erectile dysfunction (Postuma et al., 2013).

It is not clear whether RBD itself directly impacts sleep quality and structure in PD. Although some studies do not suggest this (Sixel-Doring, Trautmann et al., 2011), abnormalities in progression of REM over the night in patients with RBD compared to those without have been reported (Arnaldi, Latimier, Leu-Semenescu, Vidailhet, & Arnulf, 2016). In addition, several sleep disorders are comorbid in PD patients with RBD compared to those without including higher prevalence of nightmares, sleep talking, and restless legs syndrome (Di Fabio, Poryazova, Oberholzer, Baumann, & Bassetti, 2013; Munhoz et al., 2013; Ylikoski, Martikainen, & Partinen, 2014). As delineated in Chapter 12, PD patients with RBD are more likely to have excessive daytime sleepiness (Rolinski et al., 2014) and shortened sleep latency (Plomhause et al., 2013). In addition, PD patients with RBD are more likely to have sleep onset insomnia (see also Chapter 1), sleep maintenance insomnia (see also Chapter 2), and early morning awakening (Poryazova, Oberholzer, Baumann, & Bassetti, 2013; Suzuki et al., 2013; Vibha et al., 2011).

A meta-analysis examining differences in PD patients with RBD compared to those without included 31 articles with data from 5785 patients (with either pRBD or RBD). This study confirmed increased odds of RBD in males with longer disease duration, higher Hoehn and Yahr, and higher motor score (Zhu et al., 2017).

Management

There is a high risk of sleep-related injury to patients and their bed partners, resulting from dream enactment (Devnani & Fernandes, 2015; Olson, Boeve, & Silber, 2000). This may be especially true for patients with vivid dream recall (McCarter, St Louis, Boswell et al., 2014). Pharmacotherapy is indicated to help reduce this risk, but instituting nonpharmacologic safety measures is a critical part of the management of RBD in PD as well (Devnani & Fernandes, 2015). There are no data to support which safety measures are most effective and the following recommendations are based on common sense and/or anecdotal reports. Simple measures include moving furniture, especially a bedside table, away from the bed, or at least padding its corners and rim (such as with materials used for "baby-proofing" the room). Padding of any firm headboards is important as well. Placement of long "body pillows" between the patient and their bed partner could reduce risk of injury to the bed partner. In instances where dream enactment is frequent and violent, it may be safest to have the patient sleep on a mattress placed directly on the floor. Some patients instead sleep in a sleeping bag, placed on their bed, to protect themselves and their bed partner. Bed alarms have been reported of use in a small case series.

There are few data to guide pharmacotherapy of RBD in PD. In the idiopathic RBD (iRBD) population, clonazepam and melatonin are the mainstays of therapy (Aurora et al., 2010). Melatonin has a demonstrated polysomnographic effect to reduce the degree of RWA and this translates clinically to reduced frequency of RBD episodes (Kunz & Mahlberg, 2010). In the treatment of RBD in PD, melatonin and clonazepam are first line agents based on extension of data from iRBD and the few data from PD samples (de Almeida, Pachito, Sobreira-Neto, Tumas, & Eckeli, 2018). In PD, melatonin and clonazepam are considered to have a level of quality of evidence B: low-level quality randomized clinical trials or high quality case cohort studies (Devnani & Fernandes, 2015). However, this is with the understanding that both safety and efficacy data in PD, a population considered vulnerable to adverse effects especially of sedating medications, are limited. An open-label study of Ramelteon, a melatonin receptor agonist, indicated that it may also be useful for RBD and other sleep disturbances in PD (Kashihara et al., 2016), but additional studies on it are needed.

The impact of dopaminergic therapy on RBD is mixed; some patients have an improvement in dream enactment, whereas in other patients, dopaminergic therapy triggers or exacerbates dream enactment (Devnani & Fernandes, 2015). In a cohort of 98 patients with idiopathic RBD, pramipexole improved dream enactment and improved percent of REM sleep spent with atonia (Sasai, Matsuura, & Inoue, 2013), but to what degree this extends to RBD in PD is not clear.

Acetylcholine esterase inhibitors can cause vivid dreams and may precipitate or exacerbate RBD. However, pilot data indicate that acetylcholine esterase inhibitors, namely rivastigmine, may also be useful for RBD in PD as well, reducing the number of dream enactment episodes in small studies (de Almeida et al., 2018; Di Giacopo et al., 2012). Memantine has also been reported in small pilot studies to reduce probable dream enactment (Olin, Aarsland, & Meng, 2010), but its side effects, including daytime sedation, may limit its use in PD (de Almeida et al., 2018).

Illustrative case in context

The case is of a 69-year-old man with Parkinson's disease who sustained injury during a presumed dream enactment episode. The patient's dream recall may indicate a higher risk of injury. Mirtazapine can precipitate or exacerbate dream enactment episodes and its substitution with an antidepressant that can be dosed in the morning is indicated. Institution of safety measures is critical to reducing risk of injury. This includes removing all unnecessary furniture from around the bed, padding any remaining bedside tables, the headboard, and floor next to the bed. Melatonin is indicated to reduce dream enactment episodes and if they persist, and especially if risk of injury remains a concern, clonazepam may be indicated as well, despite his age.

References

de Almeida, C. M. O., Pachito, D. V., Sobreira-Neto, M. A., Tumas, V., & Eckeli, A. L. (2018). Pharmacological treatment for REM sleep behavior disorder in Parkinson disease and related conditions: A scoping review. *Journal of the Neurological Sciences, 393*, 63–68.

American Academy of Sleep Medicine. (2014). *International classification of sleep disorders* (3rd ed.). Darien, IL: American Academy of Sleep Medicine.

American Academy of Sleep Medicine. (April 2018). *The AASM manual for the scoring of sleep and associated events: Rules, terminology and technical specifications.*

Anang, J. B., Gagnon, J. F., Bertrand, J. A., Romenets, S. R., Latreille, V., Panisset, M., et al. (2014). Predictors of dementia in Parkinson disease: A prospective cohort study. *Neurology, 83*(14), 1253–1260.

Arnaldi, D., Latimier, A., Leu-Semenescu, S., Vidailhet, M., & Arnulf, I. (2016). Loss of REM sleep features across nighttime in REM sleep behavior disorder. *Sleep Medicine, 17*, 134–137.

Aurora, R. N., Zak, R. S., Maganti, R. K., Auerbach, S. H., Casey, K. R., Chowdhuri, S., et al. (2010). Best practice guide for the treatment of REM sleep behavior disorder (RBD). *Journal of Clinical Sleep Medicine: Official Publication of the American Academy of Sleep Medicine, 6*(1), 85–95.

Aygun, D., Turkel, Y., Onar, M. K., & Sunter, T. (2014). Clinical REM sleep behavior disorder and motor subtypes in Parkinson's disease: A questionnaire-based study. *Clinical Neurology and Neurosurgery, 119*, 54–58.

Bargiotas, P., Ntafouli, M., Lachenmayer, M. L., Krack, P., Schupbach, W. M. M., & Bassetti, C. L. A. (2019). Apathy in Parkinson's disease with REM sleep behavior disorder. *Journal of the Neurological Sciences, 399*, 194–198.

Bellosta Diago, E., Lopez Del Val, L. J., Santos Lasaosa, S., Lopez Garcia, E., & Viloria Alebesque, A. (2017). Association between REM sleep behaviour disorder and impulse control disorder in patients with Parkinson's disease [Relacion entre el trastorno de conducta del sueno REM y el trastorno de control de impulsos en pacientes con enfermedad de Parkinson]. *Neurologia, 32*(8), 494–499.

Benninger, D. H., Michel, J., Waldvogel, D., Candia, V., Poryazova, R., van Hedel, H. J., et al. (2010). REM sleep behavior disorder is not linked to postural instability and gait dysfunction in Parkinson. *Movement Disorders: Official Journal of the Movement Disorder Society, 25*(11), 1597–1604.

Bjornara, K. A., Dietrichs, E., & Toft, M. (2013). REM sleep behavior disorder in Parkinson's disease–is there a gender difference? *Parkinsonism & Related Disorders, 19*(1), 120–122.

Bjornara, K. A., Dietrichs, E., & Toft, M. (2015). Longitudinal assessment of probable rapid eye movement sleep behaviour disorder in Parkinson's disease. *European Journal of Neurology, 22*(8), 1242–1244.

Bjornara, K. A., Pihlstrom, L., Dietrichs, E., & Toft, M. (2018). Risk variants of the alpha-synuclein locus and REM sleep behavior disorder in Parkinson's disease: A genetic association study. *BMC Neurology, 18*(1), 20-2018-1023-6.

Boeve, B. F., Molano, J. R., Ferman, T. J., Smith, G. E., Lin, S. C., Bieniek, K., et al. (2011). Validation of the Mayo Sleep Questionnaire to screen for REM sleep behavior disorder in an aging and dementia cohort. *Sleep Medicine, 12*(5), 445–453.

Boeve, B. F., Silber, M. H., Saper, C. B., Ferman, T. J., Dickson, D. W., Parisi, J. E., et al. (2007). Pathophysiology of REM sleep behaviour disorder and relevance to neurodegenerative disease. *Brain: A Journal of Neurology, 130*(Pt 11), 2770−2788.

Bolitho, S. J., Naismith, S. L., Terpening, Z., Grunstein, R. R., Melehan, K., Yee, B. J., et al. (2014). Investigating rapid eye movement sleep without atonia in Parkinson's disease using the rapid eye movement sleep behavior disorder screening questionnaire. *Movement Disorders: Official Journal of the Movement Disorder Society, 29*(6), 736−742.

Bugalho, P., & Viana-Baptista, M. (2013). REM sleep behavior disorder and motor dysfunction in Parkinson's disease − a longitudinal study. *Parkinsonism & Related Disorders*.

Chahine, L. M., Daley, J., Horn, S., Colcher, A., Hurtig, H., Cantor, C., et al. (2013). Questionnaire-based diagnosis of REM sleep behavior disorder in Parkinson's disease. *Movement Disorders: Official Journal of the Movement Disorder Society, 28*(8), 1146−1149.

Chahine, L. M., Xie, S. X., Simuni, T., Tran, B., Postuma, R., Amara, A., et al. (2016). Longitudinal changes in cognition in early Parkinson's disease patients with REM sleep behavior disorder. *Parkinsonism & Related Disorders*.

Chung, S. J., Lee, Y., Lee, J. J., Lee, P. H., & Sohn, Y. H. (2017). Rapid eye movement sleep behaviour disorder and striatal dopamine depletion in patients with Parkinson's disease. *European Journal of Neurology, 24*(10), 1314−1319.

De Cock, V. C., Vidailhet, M., Leu, S., Texeira, A., Apartis, E., Elbaz, A., et al. (2007). Restoration of normal motor control in Parkinson's disease during REM sleep. *Brain: A Journal of Neurology, 130*(Pt 2), 450−456.

Devnani, P., & Fernandes, R. (2015). Management of REM sleep behavior disorder: An evidence based review. *Annals of Indian Academy of Neurology, 18*(1), 1−5.

Di Fabio, N., Poryazova, R., Oberholzer, M., Baumann, C. R., & Bassetti, C. L. (2013). Sleepwalking, REM sleep behaviour disorder and overlap parasomnia in patients with Parkinson's disease. *European Neurology, 70*(5−6), 297−303.

Di Giacopo, R., Fasano, A., Quaranta, D., Della Marca, G., Bove, F., & Bentivoglio, A. R. (2012). Rivastigmine as alternative treatment for refractory REM behavior disorder in Parkinson's disease. *Movement Disorders: Official Journal of the Movement Disorder Society, 27*(4), 559−561.

Duarte Folle, A., Paul, K. C., Bronstein, J. M., Keener, A. M., & Ritz, B. (2019). Clinical progression in Parkinson's disease with features of REM sleep behavior disorder: A population-based longitudinal study. *Parkinsonism & Related Disorders*.

Ferri, R., Fulda, S., Cosentino, F. I., Pizza, F., & Plazzi, G. (2012). A preliminary quantitative analysis of REM sleep chin EMG in Parkinson's disease with or without REM sleep behavior disorder. *Sleep Medicine, 13*(6), 707−713.

Forsaa, E. B., Larsen, J. P., Wentzel-Larsen, T., Goetz, C. G., Stebbins, G. T., Aarsland, D., et al. (2010). A 12-year population-based study of psychosis in Parkinson disease. *Archives of Neurology, 67*(8), 996−1001.

Frauscher, B., Iranzo, A., Gaig, C., Gschliesser, V., Guaita, M., Raffelseder, V., et al. (2012). Normative EMG values during REM sleep for the diagnosis of REM sleep behavior disorder. *Sleep, 35*(6), 835−847.

Frauscher, B., Jennum, P., Ju, Y. E., Postuma, R. B., Arnulf, I., Cochen De Cock, V., et al. (2014). Comorbidity and medication in REM sleep behavior disorder: A multicenter case-control study. *Neurology, 82*(12), 1076−1079.

Gagnon, J. F., Fantini, M. L., Bedard, M. A., Petit, D., Carrier, J., Rompre, S., et al. (2004). Association between waking EEG slowing and REM sleep behavior disorder in PD without dementia. *Neurology, 62*(3), 401−406.

Gagnon, J. F., Vendette, M., Postuma, R. B., Desjardins, C., Massicotte-Marquez, J., Panisset, M., et al. (2009). Mild cognitive impairment in rapid eye movement sleep behavior disorder and Parkinson's disease. *Annals of Neurology, 66*(1), 39−47.

Gaig, C., Iranzo, A., Pujol, M., Perez, H., & Santamaria, J. (2017). Periodic Limb Movements During Sleep Mimicking REM Sleep Behavior Disorder: A New Form of Periodic Limb Movement Disorder. *Sleep, 40*(3).

Garcia-Lorenzo, D., Longo-Dos Santos, C., Ewenczyk, C., Leu-Semenescu, S., Gallea, C., Quattrocchi, G., et al. (2013). The coeruleus/subcoeruleus complex in rapid eye movement sleep behaviour disorders in Parkinson's disease. *Brain: A Journal of Neurology, 136*(Pt 7), 2120−2129.

Gaudreault, P. O., Gagnon, J. F., Montplaisir, J., Vendette, M., Postuma, R. B., Gagnon, K., et al. (2013). Abnormal occipital event-related potentials in Parkinson's disease with concomitant REM sleep behavior disorder. *Parkinsonism & Related Disorders, 19*(2), 212−217.

Gong, Y., Xiong, K. P., Mao, C. J., Shen, Y., Hu, W. D., Huang, J. Y., et al. (2014). Clinical manifestations of Parkinson disease and the onset of rapid eye movement sleep behavior disorder. *Sleep Medicine, 15*(6), 647−653.

Halsband, C., Zapf, A., Sixel-Doring, F., Trenkwalder, C., & Mollenhauer, B. (2018). The REM sleep behavior disorder screening questionnaire is not valid in de Novo Parkinson's disease. *Movement Disorders Clinical Practice, 5*(2), 171−176.

Iranzo, A., & Santamaria, J. (2005). Severe obstructive sleep apnea/hypopnea mimicking REM sleep behavior disorder. *Sleep, 28*(2), 203−206.

Jozwiak, N., Postuma, R. B., Montplaisir, J., Latreille, V., Panisset, M., Chouinard, S., et al. (2017). REM sleep behavior disorder and cognitive impairment in Parkinson's disease. *Sleep, 40*(8). https://doi.org/10.1093/sleep/zsx101.

Kamps, S., van den Heuvel, O. A., van der Werf, Y. D., Berendse, H. W., Weintraub, D., & Vriend, C. (2018). Smaller subcortical volume in Parkinson patients with rapid eye movement sleep behavior disorder. *Brain Imaging and Behavior*.

Kashihara, K., Nomura, T., Maeda, T., Tsuboi, Y., Mishima, T., Takigawa, H., et al. (2016). Beneficial effects of Ramelteon on rapid eye movement sleep behavior disorder associated with Parkinson's disease − results of a multicenter open trial. *Internal Medicine, 55*(3), 231−236.

Kempfner, J., Sorensen, G., Zoetmulder, M., Jennum, P., & Sorensen, H. B. (2010). REM behaviour disorder detection associated with neurodegenerative diseases. In *Conference proceedings: Annual international conference of the IEEE Engineering in Medicine and Biology Society* (pp. 5093−5096).

Kim, J. S., Park, H. E., Oh, Y. S., Lee, S. H., Park, J. W., Son, B. C., et al. (2016). Orthostatic hypotension and cardiac sympathetic denervation in Parkinson disease patients with REM sleep behavioral disorder. *Journal of the Neurological Sciences, 362*, 59−63.

Kim, Y. E., Yang, H. J., Yun, J. Y., Kim, H. J., Lee, J. Y., & Jeon, B. S. (2014). REM sleep behavior disorder in Parkinson disease: Association with abnormal ocular motor findings. *Parkinsonism & Related Disorders, 20*(4), 444−446.

Kotagal, V., Albin, R. L., Muller, M. L., Koeppe, R. A., Chervin, R. D., Frey, K. A., et al. (2012). Symptoms of rapid eye movement sleep behavior disorder are associated with cholinergic denervation in Parkinson disease. *Annals of Neurology, 71*(4), 560−568.

Kumru, H., Santamaria, J., Tolosa, E., & Iranzo, A. (2007). Relation between subtype of Parkinson's disease and REM sleep behavior disorder. *Sleep Medicine, 8*(7−8), 779−783.

Kunz, D., & Mahlberg, R. (2010). A two-part, double-blind, placebo-controlled trial of exogenous melatonin in REM sleep behaviour disorder. *Journal of Sleep Research, 19*(4), 591−596.

Li, D., Huang, P., Zang, Y., Lou, Y., Cen, Z., Gu, Q., et al. (2017). Abnormal baseline brain activity in Parkinson's disease with and without REM sleep behavior disorder: A resting-state functional MRI study. *Journal of Magnetic Resonance Imaging: JMRI, 46*(3), 697−703.

Li, K., Li, S. H., Su, W., & Chen, H. B. (2017). Diagnostic accuracy of REM sleep behaviour disorder screening questionnaire: A meta-analysis. *Neurological Sciences: Official Journal of the Italian Neurological Society and of the Italian Society of Clinical Neurophysiology, 38*(6), 1039−1046.

Liu, H., Ou, R., Wei, Q., Hou, Y., Cao, B., Zhao, B., et al. (2019). Rapid eye movement behavior disorder in drug-naive patients with Parkinson's disease. *Journal of Clinical Neuroscience: Official Journal of the Neurosurgical Society of Australasia, 59,* 254−258.

Liu, Y., Zhu, X. Y., Zhang, X. J., Kuo, S. H., Ondo, W. G., & Wu, Y. C. (2017). Clinical features of Parkinson's disease with and without rapid eye movement sleep behavior disorder. *Translational Neurodegeneration, 6,* 35, 3017-0105-5. eCollection 2017.

Louter, M., Arends, J. B., Bloem, B. R., & Overeem, S. (2014). Actigraphy as a diagnostic aid for REM sleep behavior disorder in Parkinson's disease. *BMC Neurology, 14,* 76, 2377-14-76.

Mahale, R. R., Yadav, R., & Pal, P. K. (2016). Rapid eye movement sleep behaviour disorder in women with Parkinson's disease is an underdiagnosed entity. *Journal of Clinical Neuroscience: Official Journal of the Neurosurgical Society of Australasia, 28,* 43−46.

Manni, R., Terzaghi, M., Repetto, A., Zangaglia, R., & Pacchetti, C. (2010 Jun 15). Complex paroxysmal nocturnal behaviors in Parkinson's disease. *Movement Disorders: Official Journal of the Movement Disorder Society, 25*(8), 985−990.

Marques, A., Dujardin, K., Boucart, M., Pins, D., Delliaux, M., Defebvre, L., et al. (2010). REM sleep behaviour disorder and visuoperceptive dysfunction: A disorder of the ventral visual stream? *Journal of Neurology, 257*(3), 383−391.

Mayer, G., Bitterlich, M., Kuwert, T., Ritt, P., & Stefan, H. (2015). Ictal SPECT in patients with rapid eye movement sleep behaviour disorder. *Brain: A Journal of Neurology, 138*(Pt 5), 1263−1270.

McCarter, S. J., St Louis, E. K., Boswell, C. L., Dueffert, L. G., Slocumb, N., Boeve, B. F., et al. (2014). Factors associated with injury in REM sleep behavior disorder. *Sleep Medicine, 15*(11), 1332−1338.

McCarter, S. J., St Louis, E. K., Duwell, E. J., Timm, P. C., Sandness, D. J., Boeve, B. F., et al. (2014). Diagnostic thresholds for quantitative REM sleep phasic burst duration, phasic and tonic muscle activity, and REM atonia index in REM sleep behavior disorder with and without comorbid obstructive sleep apnea. *Sleep, 37*(10), 1649−1662.

Montplaisir, J., Gagnon, J. F., Fantini, M. L., Postuma, R. B., Dauvilliers, Y., Desautels, A., et al. (2010). Polysomnographic diagnosis of idiopathic REM sleep behavior disorder. *Movement Disorders: Official Journal of the Movement Disorder Society, 25*(13), 2044−2051.

Munhoz, R. P., Teive, H. A., Eleftherohorinou, H., Coin, L. J., Lees, A. J., & Silveira-Moriyama, L. (2013). Demographic and motor features associated with the occurrence of neuropsychiatric and sleep complications of Parkinson's disease. *Journal of Neurology, Neurosurgery & Psychiatry, 84*(8), 883−887.

Neikrug, A. B., Maglione, J. E., Liu, L., Natarajan, L., Avanzino, J. A., Corey-Bloom, J., et al. (2013). Effects of sleep disorders on the non-motor symptoms of Parkinson disease. *Journal of Clinical Sleep Medicine: Official Publication of the American Academy of Sleep Medicine, 9*(11), 1119−1129.

Nihei, Y., Takahashi, K., Koto, A., Mihara, B., Morita, Y., Isozumi, K., et al. (2012). REM sleep behavior disorder in Japanese patients with Parkinson's disease: A multicenter study using the REM sleep behavior disorder screening questionnaire. *Journal of Neurology, 259*(8), 1606−1612.

Nomura, T., Inoue, Y., Kagimura, T., Uemura, Y., & Nakashima, K. (2011). Utility of the REM sleep behavior disorder screening questionnaire (RBDSQ) in Parkinson's disease patients. *Sleep Medicine, 12*(7), 711−713.

Nomura, T., Kishi, M., & Nakashima, K. (2017). Differences in clinical characteristics when REM sleep behavior disorder precedes or comes after the onset of Parkinson's disease. *Journal of the Neurological Sciences, 382*, 58−60.

Olin, J. T., Aarsland, D., & Meng, X. (2010). Rivastigmine in the treatment of dementia associated with Parkinson's disease: Effects on activities of daily living. *Dementia and Geriatric Cognitive Disorders, 29*(6), 510−515.

Olson, E. J., Boeve, B. F., & Silber, M. H. (2000). Rapid eye movement sleep behaviour disorder: Demographic, clinical and laboratory findings in 93 cases. *Brain: A Journal of Neurology, 123*(Pt 2), 331−339.

Pacchetti, C., Manni, R., Zangaglia, R., Mancini, F., Marchioni, E., Tassorelli, C., et al. (2005). Relationship between hallucinations, delusions, and rapid eye movement sleep behavior disorder in Parkinson's disease. *Movement Disorders: Official Journal of the Movement Disorder Society, 20*(11), 1439−1448.

Pagano, G., De Micco, R., Yousaf, T., Wilson, H., Chandra, A., & Politis, M. (2018). REM behavior disorder predicts motor progression and cognitive decline in Parkinson disease. *Neurology, 91*(10), e894−e905.

Parkkinen, L., Pirttila, T., & Alafuzoff, I. (2008). Applicability of current staging/categorization of alpha-synuclein pathology and their clinical relevance. *Acta Neuropathologica, 115*(4), 399−407.

Plomhause, L., Dujardin, K., Boucart, M., Herlin, V., Defebvre, L., Derambure, P., et al. (2014). Impaired visual perception in rapid eye movement sleep behavior disorder. *Neuropsychology, 28*(3), 388−393.

Plomhause, L., Dujardin, K., Duhamel, A., Delliaux, M., Derambure, P., Defebvre, L., et al. (2013). Rapid eye movement sleep behavior disorder in treatment-naive Parkinson disease patients. *Sleep Medicine.*

Poryazova, R., Oberholzer, M., Baumann, C. R., & Bassetti, C. L. (2013). REM sleep behavior disorder in Parkinson's disease: A questionnaire-based survey. *Journal of Clinical Sleep Medicine: Official Publication of the American Academy of Sleep Medicine, 9*(1), 55−59.

Postuma, R. B., Arnulf, I., Hogl, B., Iranzo, A., Miyamoto, T., Dauvilliers, Y., et al. (2012). A single-question screen for rapid eye movement sleep behavior disorder: A multicenter validation study. *Movement Disorders: Official Journal of the Movement Disorder Society, 27*(7), 913−916.

Postuma, R. B., Bertrand, J. A., Montplaisir, J., Desjardins, C., Vendette, M., Rios Romenets, S., et al. (2012). Rapid eye movement sleep behavior disorder and risk of dementia in Parkinson's disease: A prospective study. *Movement Disorders: Official Journal of the Movement Disorder Society, 27*(6), 720−726.

Postuma, R. B., Gagnon, J. F., Pelletier, A., & Montplaisir, J. (2013). Prodromal autonomic symptoms and signs in Parkinson's disease and dementia with Lewy bodies. *Movement Disorders: Official Journal of the Movement Disorder Society, 28*(5), 597–604.

Postuma, R. B., Gagnon, J. F., Vendette, M., Charland, K., & Montplaisir, J. (2008a). Manifestations of Parkinson disease differ in association with REM sleep behavior disorder. *Movement Disorders: Official Journal of the Movement Disorder Society, 23*(12), 1665–1672.

Postuma, R. B., Gagnon, J. F., Vendette, M., Charland, K., & Montplaisir, J. (2008b). REM sleep behaviour disorder in Parkinson's disease is associated with specific motor features. *Journal of Neurology, Neurosurgery & Psychiatry, 79*(10), 1117–1121.

Postuma, R. B., Lanfranchi, P. A., Blais, H., Gagnon, J. F., & Montplaisir, J. Y. (2010). Cardiac autonomic dysfunction in idiopathic REM sleep behavior disorder. *Movement Disorders: Official Journal of the Movement Disorder Society, 25*(14), 2304–2310.

Postuma, R. B., Montplaisir, J., Lanfranchi, P., Blais, H., Rompre, S., Colombo, R., et al. (2011). Cardiac autonomic denervation in Parkinson's disease is linked to REM sleep behavior disorder. *Movement Disorders: Official Journal of the Movement Disorder Society, 26*(8), 1529–1533.

Rolinski, M., Szewczyk-Krolikowski, K., Tomlinson, P. R., Nithi, K., Talbot, K., Ben-Shlomo, Y., et al. (2014). REM sleep behaviour disorder is associated with worse quality of life and other non-motor features in early Parkinson's disease. *Journal of Neurology, Neurosurgery & Psychiatry, 85*(5), 560–566.

Romenets, S. R., Gagnon, J. F., Latreille, V., Panniset, M., Chouinard, S., Montplaisir, J., et al. (2012). Rapid eye movement sleep behavior disorder and subtypes of Parkinson's disease. *Movement Disorders: Official Journal of the Movement Disorder Society.*

Salsone, M., Cerasa, A., Arabia, G., Morelli, M., Gambardella, A., Mumoli, L., et al. (2014). Reduced thalamic volume in Parkinson disease with REM sleep behavior disorder: Volumetric study. *Parkinsonism & Related Disorders, 20*(9), 1004–1008.

Sasai, T., Matsuura, M., & Inoue, Y. (2013). Factors associated with the effect of pramipexole on symptoms of idiopathic REM sleep behavior disorder. *Parkinsonism & Related Disorders, 19*(2), 153–157.

Shen, S. S., Shen, Y., Xiong, K. P., Chen, J., Mao, C. J., Huang, J. Y., et al. (2014). Validation study of REM sleep behavior disorder questionnaire-Hong Kong (RBDQ-HK) in east China. *Sleep Medicine, 15*(8), 952–958.

Sinforiani, E., Pacchetti, C., Zangaglia, R., Pasotti, C., Manni, R., & Nappi, G. (2008). REM behavior disorder, hallucinations and cognitive impairment in Parkinson's disease: A two-year follow up. *Movement Disorders: Official Journal of the Movement Disorder Society, 23*(10), 1441–1445.

Sinforiani, E., Zangaglia, R., Manni, R., Cristina, S., Marchioni, E., Nappi, G., et al. (2006). REM sleep behavior disorder, hallucinations, and cognitive impairment in Parkinson's disease. *Movement Disorders: Official Journal of the Movement Disorder Society, 21*(4), 462–466.

Sixel-Doring, F., Schweitzer, M., Mollenhauer, B., & Trenkwalder, C. (2011). Intraindividual variability of REM sleep behavior disorder in Parkinson's disease: A comparative assessment using a new REM sleep behavior disorder severity scale (RBDSS) for clinical routine. *Journal of Clinical Sleep Medicine: Official Publication of the American Academy of Sleep Medicine, 7*(1), 75–80.

Sixel-Doring, F., Trautmann, E., Mollenhauer, B., & Trenkwalder, C. (2011). Associated factors for REM sleep behavior disorder in Parkinson disease. *Neurology, 77*(11), 1048−1054.

Sixel-Doring, F., Trautmann, E., Mollenhauer, B., & Trenkwalder, C. (2012). Age, drugs, or disease: What alters the macrostructure of sleep in Parkinson's disease? *Sleep Medicine, 13*(9), 1178−1183.

Sixel-Doring, F., Trautmann, E., Mollenhauer, B., & Trenkwalder, C. (2014). Rapid eye movement sleep behavioral events: A new marker for neurodegeneration in early Parkinson disease? *Sleep, 37*(3), 431−438.

Sommerauer, M., Valko, P. O., Werth, E., Poryazova, R., Hauser, S., & Baumann, C. R. (2014). Revisiting the impact of REM sleep behavior disorder on motor progression in Parkinson's disease. *Parkinsonism & Related Disorders, 20*(4), 460−464.

Stefani, A., Mahlknecht, P., Seppi, K., Nocker, M., Mair, K. J., Hotter, A., et al. (2016). Consistency of "probable RBD" diagnosis with the RBD screening questionnaire: A follow-up study. *Movement Disorders Clinical Practice, 4*(3), 403−405.

Stiasny-Kolster, K., Mayer, G., Schafer, S., Moller, J. C., Heinzel-Gutenbrunner, M., & Oertel, W. H. (2007). The REM sleep behavior disorder screening questionnaire–a new diagnostic instrument. *Movement Disorders: Official Journal of the Movement Disorder Society, 22*(16), 2386−2393.

Stiasny-Kolster, K., Sixel-Doring, F., Trenkwalder, C., Heinzel-Gutenbrunner, M., Seppi, K., Poewe, W., et al. (2015). Diagnostic value of the REM sleep behavior disorder screening questionnaire in Parkinson's disease. *Sleep Medicine, 16*(1), 186−189.

Suzuki, K., Miyamoto, T., Miyamoto, M., Watanabe, Y., Suzuki, S., Tatsumoto, M., et al. (2013). Probable rapid eye movement sleep behavior disorder, nocturnal disturbances and quality of life in patients with Parkinson's disease: A case-controlled study using the rapid eye movement sleep behavior disorder screening questionnaire. *BMC Neurology, 13*, 18, 2377-13-18.

Terzaghi, M., Arnaldi, D., Rizzetti, M. C., Minafra, B., Cremascoli, R., Rustioni, V., et al. (2013). Analysis of video-polysomnographic sleep findings in dementia with Lewy bodies. *Movement Disorders: Official Journal of the Movement Disorder Society, 28*(10), 1416−1423.

Vendette, M., Gagnon, J. F., Decary, A., Massicotte-Marquez, J., Postuma, R. B., Doyon, J., et al. (2007). REM sleep behavior disorder predicts cognitive impairment in Parkinson disease without dementia. *Neurology, 69*(19), 1843−1849.

Vibha, D., Shukla, G., Goyal, V., Singh, S., Srivastava, A. K., & Behari, M. (2011). RBD in Parkinson's disease: A clinical case control study from North India. *Clinical Neurology and Neurosurgery, 113*(6), 472−476.

Ylikoski, A., Martikainen, K., & Partinen, M. (2014). Parasomnias and isolated sleep symptoms in Parkinson's disease: A questionnaire study on 661 patients. *Journal of the Neurological Sciences, 346*(1−2), 204−208.

Zhu, R. L., Xie, C. J., Hu, P. P., & Wang, K. (2017). Clinical variations in Parkinson's disease patients with or without REM sleep behaviour disorder: A meta-analysis. *Scientific Reports, 7*, 40779.

Zibetti, M., Rizzi, L., Colloca, L., Cinquepalmi, A., Angrisano, S., Castelli, L., et al. (2010). Probable REM sleep behaviour disorder and STN-DBS outcome in Parkinson's disease. *Parkinsonism & Related Disorders, 16*(4), 265−269.

REM sleep behavior disorder as a prodromal Parkinson's disease feature

Illustrative case

A 65-year-old man presents, accompanied by his wife, to the outpatient Sleep Disorders Clinic with "restless sleep." They report that he has had episodes in which he has kicked, punched, and even strangled his wife during sleep and yelled out, often cursing. He sometimes has woken himself up punching out into the air. Once he fell out of bed and recalls that in his dream he was being attacked and was running away from the assailant. He has frequent recollection of his dreams and describes them as often involving him being attacked. His wife is so scared of these episodes, and she has started to sleep in a separate room. The episodes began 3 years ago but have increased in frequency, occurring 3—4 times a month. He typically goes to bed around 10:30 p.m. and reads until he falls asleep, estimating this to be within 30 minutes. His wife reports that he sometimes snores gently when he is lying on his back. The dream enactment episodes happen around 3:00 a.m. Sometimes the episodes will wake him up but otherwise he generally sleeps through the night and wakes up around 6:00 a.m. feeling refreshed. He has a history of depression and 1 year ago was started on sertraline, which he takes at bedtime. He reports occasional afternoon sleepiness and sometimes takes a brief nap. On review of systems, he reports mild intermittent constipation and endorses loss of sense of smell. Otherwise he feels generally well and has no medical comorbidities. On examination, he has no evidence of slowness, stiffness, tremor, or other abnormalities.

Overview

Definition

Rapid eye movement (REM) sleep behavior disorder (RBD) is a parasomnia. Broadly, parasomnias are a category of sleep disorders marked by "undesirable physical events or experiences that occur during entry into sleep, within sleep, or during arousal from sleep" and that "encompass abnormal sleep related complex movements, behaviors, emotions, perceptions, dreams, and autonomic nervous system activity" (American Academy of Sleep Medicine, 2014). RBD is an REM parasomnia: a parasomnia that occurs in REM sleep. The diagnostic criteria for RBD, as defined by the American Academy of Sleep medicine, include "repeated episodes of sleep related vocalizations and/or complex motor behaviors" occurring during REM sleep (as documented on polysomnography) or based on clinical history of dream enactment. Dream enactment in RBD may range from nondescript movements such as limb jerks and unintelligible vocalizations, to more goal-directed behaviors such as gesturing, punching, or kicking. In some cases, movements commensurate with dream content may be described. For example, a patient may be dreaming of fighting off an assailant, and the dream enactment is marked by punching, yelling, and calling out for police. As in the latter example, dream content in RBD is usually action-packed and often reported as nightmares marked by violence. Behaviors and vocalizations are often out of character for the patient (for example, a normally passive or pacifistic patient may be quite physically and verbally aggressive during dream enactment episodes). However, more benign dreams and commensurate enactment behaviors such as laughing and singing may occur as well (Oudiette et al., 2009). Interestingly, patients may achieve movement amplitudes and vocalization decibels during sleep that are substantially larger/louder than their ability to move and/or vocalize during the day (De Cock, Vidailhet et al., 2007). This may be related to the bypassing of abnormal basal ganglia pathways (Mayer, Bitterlich, Kuwert, Ritt, & Stefan, 2015).

In over half of cases, patients themselves may not be aware of dream enactment episodes. Thus, ancillary information from a bed partner and/or other household members is critical. This is especially true when screening for RBD using question-naire. Validated questionnaires help screen for RBD (Stiasny-Kolster et al., 2007), but specificity and sensitivity is maximized with bed-partner input (Boeve et al., 2011).

A clinical history of dream enactment allows only for the diagnosis of possible RBD. Polysomnographic confirmation of loss of REM atonia is required for a definitive diagnosis of RBD (American Academy of Sleep Medicine, 2014). Normally during REM sleep, there is atonia, or loss of muscle activity, in most muscles (with some exceptions including the diaphragm and extraocular muscles). In RBD, REM without atonia (RWA) is documented on polysomnography as increased muscle activity seen on surface EMG electrodes placed on the chin or other areas.

(Regarding the latter, surface EMG recordings from the flexor digitorum superficialis may be particularly sensitive for capturing RWA (Frauscher, Ehrmann, & Hogl, 2012; Frauscher, Iranzo et al., 2012; Frauscher et al., 2008). However, in routine sleep lab settings, it is mainly the chin EMG that is included, and therefore the chin EMG is the main signal considered in determining RWA in most cases, especially outside of the research setting. There are two main types of increased activity defined: tonic, in which the increase in EMG activity is twice the baseline and lasts 15 seconds or more, and phasic, in which the activity is four times baseline. Normative data for age and sex that help to inform the determination of RWA, based on the percentage of REM sleep during which EMG goes above the thresholds considered abnormal, have been established (American Academy of Sleep

Medicine, 2018). In general, a single night of PSG is considered adequate to assess for RWA (Ferri et al., 2013), if the patient has at least one period of REM sleep, of sufficient duration, during the study (Zhang et al., 2008). Of note is that in the presence of suspected RBD, scoring of REM sleep needs to occur while accounting for the possibility that RWA may be present. In other words, normally atonia is part of the criteria used to designate a period of sleep as REM stage, but in the presence of suspected RBD, REM sleep is scored based only on electro-oculogram and EEG findings (Lapierre & Montplaisir, 1992; Montplaisir et al., 2010). These scoring methods are labor intensive and in routine clinical evaluation of polysomnograms may not be practical. Automated scoring methods have been developed on a research basis (Cooray et al., 2018; Frauscher, Gabelia et al., 2014; Frauscher, Jennum et al., 2014; McCarter et al., 2014), and with appropriate validation may eventually be useful for clinical sleep labs as well.

Epidemiology

Robust data on the epidemiology of RBD on the population level are not available, due to the logistical challenges of performing polysomnography on a large scale. Thus, most studies investigating RBD epidemiology are based on screening questionnaires or telephone interviews that, at best, allow for designation of "possible RBD" (see definition section). Studies using questionnaire-based screening for RBD indicate a prevalence of 3%−10% (Boot et al., 2012; C. Ma et al., 2017; J.F. Ma et al., 2017; Mahlknecht, Seppi et al., 2015; Wong et al., 2016). A few studies that applied polysomnography do inform polysomnographically confirmed RBD epidemiology.

In one study of community-dwelling adults older than 60 years old in South Korea (Kang et al., 2013), 696 individuals were invited to participate in a study aiming to assess the prevalence of subclinical RWA and RBD. Among them, 348 completed polysomnography and had three or more hours of sleep and two or more REM periods. Mean patient age was 68.4 (range 60−88). Polysomnographic records were reviewed for RWA, and those with RWA were contacted by telephone to ascertain history of dream enactment (from the patient and their bed partner). The crude prevalence of polysomnographically-assessed idiopathic RBD was 1.15%, and the age- and sex-standardized prevalence was 1.34. The crude prevalence of subclinical RWA (without a history of dream enactment) was 5.17, with an age- and sex-standardized prevalence of 4.95 (Kang et al., 2013).

Another study recruited community-dwelling adults aged 60 or older seen at one of two primary care centers in Spain (Pujol et al., 2017). RBD was screened for using a validated question, and those screening positive underwent polysomnography. Among 539, 28 (5.2%) screened positive. Of the 24 of those who went on to have polysomnography, an RBD mimic was found in 11: 2 had periodic limb movements, 9 had OSA. Four individuals had RWA and thus met criteria for idiopathic RBD, yielding a point prevalence of 0.74% (Pujol et al., 2017). Because, as mentioned, many patients do not recognize their dream enactment symptoms, this study may have underestimated prevalence of RBD, as mandatory bed-partner input was not part of the screening protocol.

One of the largest studies on polysomnographically confirmed RBD epidemiology was performed on the HypnoLaus study cohort (Haba-Rubio et al., 2017). HypnoLaus is a population-based study in Switzerland. Polysomnographic data (in-home studies) were available on 1977 participants, mean age 59. History of RBD was ascertained via a parasomnia-screening questionnaire: 386 participants scored positive on the questionnaires and 21 had evidence of REM sleep without atonia on the PSG. The estimated prevalence was thus 1.06%. No sex difference in prevalence was observed.

In summary, the prevalence of polysomnographically confirmed RBD in community-dwelling adults is at least 1%, and the prevalence of RWA is higher, as expected, at about 5%.

Most community-based studies on the epidemiology of RBD have not found differences in prevalence among the sexes (Haba-Rubio et al., 2017; Kang et al., 2013; Postuma et al., 2012; Wong et al., 2016). However, some studies have suggested that there may be sex differences in older individuals, where males may have a higher prevalence. Whether male sex is a risk factor for RBD or simply is associated with patient characteristics that increase detection/diagnosis of RBD is not clear (Teman, Tippmann-Peikert, Silber, Slocumb, & Auger, 2009). Age is the other major risk factor for RBD (Haba-Rubio et al., 2017; Kang et al., 2013; Postuma et al., 2012; Wong et al., 2016). As for other risk factors, as discussed further later, most patients with idiopathic RBD go on to develop a synucleinopathy: a neurodegenerative parkinsonian disorder marked pathologically by the presence of abnormal α-synuclein. These disorders including Parkinson's disease (PD), dementia with Lewy bodies, and multiple system atrophy. It is not surprising, therefore, that the environmental risk factors for RBD are also risk factors for PD, namely pesticide exposure and history of head trauma (Frauscher, Gabelia et al., 2014; Frauscher, Jennum et al., 2014; Postuma et al., 2012). It is also not surprising that specific single nucleotide polymorphisms in genes related to increased risk of PD are associated with increased risk of RBD as well (Gan-Or et al., 2015, 2017; Pont-Sunyer et al., 2015).

Etiology and differential diagnosis

Data from animals and humans indicate that RBD results from involvement of specific pathways in the brainstem, involving several neurotransmitter systems (Boeve et al., 2007; Garcia-Lorenzo et al., 2013; Kim et al., 2014). These pathways are still to be fully elucidated. REM without atonia may be generated in part from lesions in the sublaterodorsal nucleus of the rat, which corresponds to the glutamatergic perilocus coeruleus in humans. GABA-ergic and glycine neurons in the ventral medulla are also involved: the ventral medulla contains the nucleus raphe magnus, the ventral and lateral gigantocellular and lateral paragigantocellular reticular nuclei that project directly to spinal motor neurons. It is inhibition of spinal motor neurons by projections from the latter nuclei that normally lead to atonia during REM sleep. Other areas/neurotransmitter systems that may be involved in the manifestation of RBD include the cholinergic pedunculopontine nucleus and the laterodorsal tegmental nucleus; lesions of these regions in cats lead to abnormal activity during REM. In humans, lesions in these areas could facilitate RWA and/or dream enactment but are not considered sufficient to cause RBD in isolation. As for the areas that generate the vivid (often violent) dreams and the subsequent dream enactment, it is hypothesized that areas rostral to the medulla/pons, possibly in the midbrain, motor cortex, and even the limbic system, may be involved (though to what degree these areas are primary generators vs. are secondarily activated is not yet clear). Importantly, a small study that performed ictal SPECT on patients with idiopathic and secondary RBD demonstrated activation of the supplementary motor area and pons, with *bypassing* of the basal ganglia during dream enactment episodes (Mayer et al., 2015).

Idiopathic RBD, or RBD with no clear underlying etiology, is of relevance in relation to sleep disorders in PD because most individuals with iRBD go on to develop a neurodegenerative synucleinopathy (see "Consequences and Implications" section later). There are other rarer etiologies of RBD (Table 6.1) (Boeve et al., 2007; Dauvilliers et al., 2018; Gaig et al., 2017; Sabater et al., 2014). These should especially be considered in younger patients (those younger than age 50) and those in which the acuity and comorbid symptoms suggest a secondary etiology. Some medications, such as selective serotonin reuptake inhibitors (SSRI), may facilitate RWA in REM sleep. Whether this has implications (regarding risk of future neurodegeneration) is not clear; it is possible that the increased risk of depression and SSRI use reported in idiopathic RBD may in part be explained by the high prevalence of depression in prodromal PD (Postuma et al., 2013).

Table 6.1 Causes of REM sleep behavior disorder.

Cause	Comment
"Idiopathic" RBD	In most patients with so-called idiopathic RBD, a neurodegenerative synucleinopathy may be present.
Narcolepsy	Typically younger age group. History of other features of narcolepsy would be present, such as sleep attacks, hypnogogic hallucinations, and cataplexy
Structural lesions of the brainstem	Lesions in critical brainstem structures in the pons and midbrain, which mediate RWA and dream enactment can lead to RBD. These include but are not limited to strokes, demyelinating lesions, tumors, and traumatic brain injury
Autoimmune disorders	Sleep problems may be the presenting feature but do not occur in isolation. Encephalopathy manifesting with cognitive dysfunction, bulbar symptoms, and motor abnormalities (gait complaints, evidence of ataxia, chorea, parkinsonism) are seen

As mentioned earlier, a history of dream enactment, without polysomnographic confirmation of RWA, allows only for a diagnosis of possible RBD. The differential diagnosis for dream enactment behavior is shown in Table 6.2 (Boeve et al., 2007; Dauvilliers et al., 2018; Gaig, Iranzo, Pujol, Perez, & Santamaria, 2017; Iranzo & Santamaria, 2005).

Consequences and complications

Most patients with idiopathic RBD go on to develop a synucleinopathy: a neurodegenerative parkinsonian disorder marked pathologically the presence of abnormal α-synuclein (Boeve et al., 2013; Iranzo, Fernandez-Arcos et al., 2014; Iranzo, Stockner et al., 2014; Postuma et al., 2019). These disorders include Parkinson's disease, dementia with Lewy bodies, and multiple system atrophy (as well as some other rare disorders) (Boeve et al., 2013). Indeed, RBD is seen as a key characteristic of prodromal PD. The first large prospective study to examine the rate of conversion to neurodegenerative disorder among individuals the RBD included 174 patients with idiopathic RBD (with polysomnographic confirmation). The 5-year risk of developing a diagnosable neurodegenerative disorder was 33.1% and the 14-year cumulative was 90.4%, although the proportion of participants reaching 14-year follow-up was small (Iranzo, Fernandez-Arcos et al., 2014; Iranzo, Stockner et al., 2014). In the largest study to date, 1280 individuals with polysomnographically confirmed idiopathic RBD were followed for a mean of 4.6 years. Average age was 66.3 years and 83% were male. The 12-year conversion rate in this study was 74% (Postuma et al., 2019). The annualized rate of conversion to a neurodegenerative disorder in an individual with idiopathic RBD is estimated at 6%−8% per year (Postuma et al., 2015). Clinical progression from idiopathic RBD to a clinically

Table 6.2 Differential diagnosis of dream enactment behavior/RBD mimics.

Differential diagnosis	Key distinguishing features
NREM sleep parasomnias	Occur in earlier part of night, out of slow wave (stage 3) sleep. Usually occur in younger age groups but can be seen in adults.
Nocturnal seizures	Polysomnography shows epileptiform activity; when suspicion for this is high, a full EEG montage during polysomnography is important to do.
Obstructive sleep apnea (OSA)	REM-related arousals lead to episodes that mimic RBD. Polysomnography shows preserved atonia. Treatment of the OSA may eliminate RBD.
Periodic limb movements	Periodicity and relative predominance in lower extremities as well as timing over the night help to distinguish periodic limb movements from dream enactment behaviors of RBD. Polysomnogram is required for definitive distinction between the two.

diagnosable synucleinopathy, often with associated cognitive impairment, is largely consistent with the neuropathological staging system posed by Braak (Braak et al., 2003) that posits progression of pathology from the olfactory regions and lower brainstem (medulla) up toward the pons, substantia nigra, and then the cortex (Braak et al., 2003). Although RBD has rarely been reported in neurodegenerative disorders without synuclein, such as the tauopathies progressive supranuclear palsy (Sixel-Doring, Schweitzer, Mollenhauer, & Trenkwalder, 2009) or Guadeloupian parkinsonism (De Cock, Lannuzel et al., 2007), this is exceedingly rare. A history of RBD in a patient with presumed tauopathy may, in fact, suggest the presence of an RBD mimic such as obstructive sleep apnea (Boeve, Silber, Ferman, Lucas, & Parisi, 2001; Iranzo & Santamaria, 2005) and deserves further evaluation (Table 6.1).

Preliminary reports indicate that RWA, even in the absence of dream enactment behavior, may be of clinical relevance (in relation to risk of future PD) (Postuma, Gagnon, Rompre, & Montplaisir, 2010; Stefani et al., 2015), but further data on this are needed.

There are no clear data to indicate that REM sleep itself, apart from the EMG changes, is abnormal in individuals with RBD compared to those without. Specifically, REM sleep latency, duration, and percent of sleep spent in REM are not clearly different in those with RBD compared to those without (Dauvilliers et al., 2018).

There are intensive efforts underway to identify biomarkers to help predict which RBD patients will go on to develop a neurodegenerative synucleinopathy, and when. Such markers will be critical for identification of high-risk patients who would benefit from preventative therapies, when they emerge. For example, immunotherapies against α-synuclein have been developed, and clinical trials could target idiopathic RBD patients with one or more markers indicating increased risk of PD. Several potential markers have been identified from clinical (Cooper & Chahine, 2016; Gagnon et al., 2009; Mahlknecht, Iranzo et al., 2015; Postuma, Gagnon, Vendette, Charland, & Montplaisir, 2008; Postuma et al., 2009; Postuma, Gagnon, Vendette, & Montplaisir, 2009a; Postuma, Gagnon, Vendette, & Montplaisir, 2009b; Postuma et al., 2019; Postuma, Lang, Massicotte-Marquez, & Montplaisir, 2006), imaging (Berg, 2009; Dang-Vu et al., 2012; Holtbernd et al., 2014; Iranzo, Fernandez-Arcos et al., 2014; Iranzo, Lomena et al., 2010; Iranzo et al., 2017; Iranzo, Stockner et al., 2014; Iranzo et al., 2011; Nomura et al., 2010; Postuma et al., 2019), electrophysiology (Fantini et al., 2003; Iranzo, Isetta et al., 2010; Postuma et al., 2010), and biofluid sources (Uribe-San Martin et al., 2013) (Table 6.3). Many still require validation in large longitudinal cohort studies. To maximize sensitivity and specificity, and accuracy regarding time to conversion, multimodal models that incorporate many different features will likely be needed (Berg et al., 2015).

RBD carries with it significant risk of injury to the patient and the bed partner. Two-thirds of bed partners reported injury in one study (Lam et al., 2016). Some severe injuries including intracerebral hemorrhage and fractures have been reported. Sadly, even deaths have occurred in the context of dream enactment from presumed

Table 6.3 Markers that may predict emergence of a neurodegenerative disorder in patients with RBD.

Category	Domain	Comment
Sensory	Olfaction	Olfactory loss is more common in RBD compared to healthy controls. Impaired olfaction predicts conversion to neurodegenerative synucleinopathy among patients with idiopathic RBD
	Vision	Impaired color vision predicted conversion to synucleinopathy
Motor	Quantitative motor testing	Abnormal testing on routinely administered clinical motor rating scales predicts conversion to neurodegenerative disorder. On a research basis, when most of the following tasks are abnormal in RBD, this predicts increased risk of conversion to neurodegenerative disorder: alternate-tap test, Purdue pegboard test, 3-m Timed-Up-and-Go test, or Flamingo balance test.
Autonomic	Cardiovascular	Orthostatic hypotension is more common in RBD compared to healthy controls and is one of the earliest prodromal symptoms seen based on patient recall. Reduced cardiac MIBG uptake is seen in RBD, but prospective studies are needed to confirm predictive value for conversion
	Genitourinary	Urinary dysfunction is more common in RBD compared to healthy controls
	Gastrointestinal	Constipation is more common in RBD compared to healthy controls
Imaging	Striatal dopaminergic deficit	Reduced dopamine transporter binding is one of the most robustly characterized markers for risk of neurodegenerative disorder in RBD.
	Substantia nigra hyperechogenicity on transcranial Doppler sonography	This ultrasound measure can maximize sensitivity of predicting conversion especially when combined with dopamine transporter imaging
	PD-related covariance pattern on PET and SPECT	A reproducible disease-related metabolic brain network, known as the PD-related covariance patter, is seen in PD. This was also found to be present in RBD and was predictive of conversion to neurodegenerative disorder
	Increased hippocampal mean regional cerebral blood flow	Hippocampal perfusion predicted conversion to a neurodegenerative disorder and was associated with other markers (color vision and motor scores)

Table 6.3 Markers that may predict emergence of a neurodegenerative disorder in patients with RBD.—*cont'd*

Category	Domain	Comment
Electrophysiology	Tonic surface EMG activity on submental EMG	Increased EMG activity in REM sleep may predict conversion to neurodegenerative disorder independent of history of dream enactment
	EEG slowing	EEG slowing during wakefulness predicts conversion to mild cognitive impairment
Biochemical	Uric acid levels	Lower uric acid levels are seen in PD compared to non-PD populations. Along these lines, higher uric acid levels are seen in those with longer duration of RBD before manifestation of PD

RBD (Fernandez-Arcos, Iranzo, Serradell, Gaig, & Santamaria, 2016; Mahowald, Bundlie, Hurwitz, & Schenck, 1990; Olson, Boeve, & Silber, 2000). It is not surprising that RBD is associated with poor quality of life for both the patient and the bed partner (Kim, Motamedi, & Cho, 2017; Lam et al., 2016). Bed-partner sleep may be disrupted both by the noise and movement occurring because of dream enactment but also by worry/fear of injury; indeed, bed partners of patients with RBD report insomnia, anxiety, and depressive symptoms (Lam et al., 2016).

Management

As mentioned, sleep-related injury may result from dream enactment episodes. Injury to both the patient and the bed partner may occur (Aurora et al., 2010; Lam et al., 2016), and one of the main goals of management is to reduce this risk of injury. Several safety measures could be recommended; these are not guided by evidence but are based on logical assumptions regarding potential risks imposed by the patient's bedroom furniture and other nighttime environmental factors. For example, any bedside lamps and bedside tables would ideally be removed where possible; an alternative is padding the edges of the bedside table. Padding firm headboards is important as well. To reduce the risk of injury to the bed partner, placing long "body pillows" between the patient and the bed partner may be recommended. Some patients sleep in sleeping bags placed on their bed. Padding the floor next to the bed (with, for example, a thick yoga matt or even a small mattress) and lowering the height of the bed (by replacing high mattresses and/or box springs) are other ideas that may be considered. Secure locks on windows, and even window alarms, may be considered.

As sleep deprivation and alcohol intake can affect REM sleep, avoiding both of these should be recommended. When comorbid OSA is present, its treatment is critical as it can reduce dream enactment episodes; care must be taken to ensure that the hose used for OSA treatment with continuous positive airway pressure does not pose risk of injury to the patient (patients could get tangled up in longer hoses). Hose holders could be considered. Finally, where possible, inciting or exacerbating medications should be addressed, such as selective serontonin reuptake inhibitors, serotonin norepinephrine reuptake inhibitors, and tricyclic antidepressants (St Louis, Boeve, & Boeve, 2017). Sometimes, moving the dosing of these medications from evening to morning can be sufficient (but this brings with it the risk of daytimes sedation for more sedating antidepressants). Obviously, switching to less sedating antidepressants is worth considering in such cases. Bupropion is one of the few antidepressants that may be associated with less risk of exacerbating dream enactment and could be considered.

Pharmacotherapy is indicated when the earlier measures do not adequately address concerns for risk of injury to either the patient or their bed partner (Aurora et al., 2010; Dauvilliers et al., 2018). Clonazepam and melatonin are the mainstays of therapy. These drugs improve frequency and severity of dream enactment behaviors. Polysomnographically, they are associated with reduced amounts muscle activity in REM (Kunz & Mahlberg, 2010; Lapierre & Montplaisir, 1992). The optimal dose of melatonin is not clear with some patients benefiting from low doses (1−3 mg) and others responding to higher doses (12−20 mg). In general, given the better safety profile of melatonin, especially in older adults, it is the preferable first line agent. Clonazepam, when necessary, should be started at the lowest possible dose and increased only gradually to effective dose. In some patients, a combination of both melatonin and clonazepam is needed to control symptoms. In all patients with RBD, lack of response to melatonin and/or clonazepam should prompt evaluation for other etiologies contributing to or exacerbating RBD (medications (see earlier discussion), obstructive sleep apnea, and alcohol intake).

There are no proven interventions to reduce risk of neurodegenerative parkinsonian disorder in patients with RBD. In the appropriate clinical context, patients may be counseled on following a generally healthy lifestyle and to be proactive to avoid head trauma (avoiding contact sports) and pesticides, as these are risk factors for Parkinson's disease. In addition, the patient may be advised that regular exercise would be prudent given its general health benefits and its possible (though unproven) neuroprotective effects. Finally, vascular risk factor modification in patients with cerebrovascular or cardiovascular history or risk factors would also be warranted.

Illustrative case in context

The case described is a 65-year-old man with a clinical history of dream enactment behavior. A polysomnogram is indicated to rule out sleep apnea, periodic limb movements, or other RBD mimics. REM without atonia (increased muscle tone during REM sleep) would confirm the diagnosis. He has no evidence of parkinsonism, but there are strong data to indicate that he is at high risk of a neurodegenerative parkinsonian disorder. Counseling on following a generally healthy lifestyle, being proactive about avoiding head trauma and pesticides, as well as regular exercise is indicated. Treatment of his depression is critical given the high risk of depression in RBD and prodromal PD. Sertraline is sedating, so switching to a less sedating antidepressant dosed in the morning, or to an antidepressant less likely to cause/exacerbate RBD (such as bupropion) may help reduce the frequency of dream enactment. Finally, safety measures should be instituted, and melatonin initiated, starting at 1 mg around 1 hour before bedtime and increasing it slowly as needed. If melatonin is insufficient to substantially reduce the frequency of dream enactment episodes, clonazepam treatment would be indicated.

References

American Academy of Sleep Medicine. (2014). *International classification of sleep disorders* (3rd ed.). Darien, IL: American Academy of Sleep Medicine.

American Academy of Sleep Medicine. (April 2018). *The AASM manual for the scoring of sleep and associated events: Rules, terminology and technical specifications.*

Aurora, R. N., Zak, R. S., Maganti, R. K., Auerbach, S. H., Casey, K. R., Chowdhuri, S., et al. (2010). Best practice guide for the treatment of REM sleep behavior disorder (RBD). *Journal of Clinical Sleep Medicine: Official Publication of the American Academy of Sleep Medicine, 6*(1), 85–95.

Berg, D. (2009). Transcranial ultrasound as a risk marker for Parkinson's disease. *Movement Disorders: Official Journal of the Movement Disorder Society, 24*(Suppl. 2), S677–S683.

Berg, D., Postuma, R. B., Adler, C. H., Bloem, B. R., Chan, P., Dubois, B., et al. (2015). MDS research criteria for prodromal Parkinson's disease. *Movement Disorders: Official Journal of the Movement Disorder Society, 30*(12), 1600–1611.

Boeve, B. F., Molano, J. R., Ferman, T. J., Smith, G. E., Lin, S. C., Bieniek, K., et al. (2011). Validation of the Mayo Sleep Questionnaire to screen for REM sleep behavior disorder in an aging and dementia cohort. *Sleep Medicine, 12*(5), 445–453.

Boeve, B. F., Silber, M. H., Ferman, T. J., Lin, S. C., Benarroch, E. E., Schmeichel, A. M., et al. (2013). Clinicopathologic correlations in 172 cases of rapid eye movement sleep behavior disorder with or without a coexisting neurologic disorder. *Sleep Medicine.*

Boeve, B. F., Silber, M. H., Ferman, T. J., Lucas, J. A., & Parisi, J. E. (2001). Association of REM sleep behavior disorder and neurodegenerative disease may reflect an underlying synucleinopathy. *Movement Disorders: Official Journal of the Movement Disorder Society, 16*(4), 622–630.

Boeve, B. F., Silber, M. H., Saper, C. B., Ferman, T. J., Dickson, D. W., Parisi, J. E., et al. (2007). Pathophysiology of REM sleep behaviour disorder and relevance to neurodegenerative disease. *Brain: A Journal of Neurology, 130*(Pt 11), 2770–2788.

Boot, B. P., Boeve, B. F., Roberts, R. O., Ferman, T. J., Geda, Y. E., Pankratz, V. S., et al. (2012). Probable rapid eye movement sleep behavior disorder increases risk for mild cognitive impairment and Parkinson disease: A population-based study. *Annals of Neurology, 71*(1), 49–56.

Braak, H., Del Tredici, K., Rub, U., de Vos, R. A., Jansen Steur, E. N., & Braak, E. (2003). Staging of brain pathology related to sporadic Parkinson's disease. *Neurobiology of Aging, 24*(2), 197–211.

Cooper, C. A., & Chahine, L. M. (2016). Biomarkers in prodromal Parkinson disease: A qualitative review. *Journal of the International Neuropsychological Society: JINS, 22*(10), 956–967.

Cooray, N., Andreotti, F., Lo, C., Symmonds, M., Hu, M. T. M., & De Vos, M. (2018). Automating the detection of REM sleep behaviour disorder. In *Conference proceedings: Annual international conference of the IEEE Engineering in Medicine and Biology Society.IEEE Engineering in Medicine and Biology Society.Annual conference, 2018* (pp. 1460–1463).

Dang-Vu, T. T., Gagnon, J. F., Vendette, M., Soucy, J. P., Postuma, R. B., & Montplaisir, J. (2012). Hippocampal perfusion predicts impending neurodegeneration in REM sleep behavior disorder. *Neurology, 79*(24), 2302–2306.

Dauvilliers, Y., Schenck, C. H., Postuma, R. B., Iranzo, A., Luppi, P. H., Plazzi, G., et al. (2018). REM sleep behaviour disorder. *Nature Reviews.Disease Primers, 4*(1), 19, 1018-0016-5.

De Cock, V. C., Lannuzel, A., Verhaeghe, S., Roze, E., Ruberg, M., Derenne, J. P., et al. (2007). REM sleep behavior disorder in patients with guadeloupean parkinsonism, a tauopathy. *Sleep, 30*(8), 1026–1032.

De Cock, V. C., Vidailhet, M., Leu, S., Texeira, A., Apartis, E., Elbaz, A., et al. (2007). Restoration of normal motor control in Parkinson's disease during REM sleep. *Brain: A Journal of Neurology, 130*(Pt 2), 450–456.

Fantini, M. L., Gagnon, J. F., Petit, D., Rompre, S., Decary, A., Carrier, J., et al. (2003). Slowing of electroencephalogram in rapid eye movement sleep behavior disorder. *Annals of Neurology, 53*(6), 774–780.

Fernandez-Arcos, A., Iranzo, A., Serradell, M., Gaig, C., & Santamaria, J. (2016). The clinical phenotype of idiopathic rapid eye movement sleep behavior disorder at presentation: A study in 203 consecutive patients. *Sleep, 39*(1), 121–132.

Ferri, R., Marelli, S., Cosentino, F. I., Rundo, F., Ferini-Strambi, L., & Zucconi, M. (2013). Night-to-night variability of automatic quantitative parameters of the chin EMG amplitude (Atonia Index) in REM sleep behavior disorder. *Journal of Clinical Sleep Medicine: Official Publication of the American Academy of Sleep Medicine, 9*(3), 253–258.

Frauscher, B., Ehrmann, L., & Hogl, B. (2012). Defining muscle activities for assessment of REM sleep behavior disorder: From a qualitative to a quantitative diagnostic level. *Sleep Medicine, 14*(8), 729–733.

Frauscher, B., Gabelia, D., Biermayr, M., Stefani, A., Hackner, H., Mitterling, T., et al. (2014). Validation of an integrated software for the detection of rapid eye movement sleep behavior disorder. *Sleep, 37*(10), 1663–1671.

Frauscher, B., Iranzo, A., Gaig, C., Gschliesser, V., Guaita, M., Raffelseder, V., et al. (2012). Normative EMG values during REM sleep for the diagnosis of REM sleep behavior disorder. *Sleep, 35*(6), 835–847.

Frauscher, B., Iranzo, A., Hogl, B., Casanova-Molla, J., Salamero, M., Gschliesser, V., et al. (2008). Quantification of electromyographic activity during REM sleep in multiple muscles in REM sleep behavior disorder. *Sleep, 31*(5), 724–731.

Frauscher, B., Jennum, P., Ju, Y. E., Postuma, R. B., Arnulf, I., Cochen De Cock, V., et al. (2014). Comorbidity and medication in REM sleep behavior disorder: A multicenter case-control study. *Neurology, 82*(12), 1076–1079.

Gagnon, J. F., Vendette, M., Postuma, R. B., Desjardins, C., Massicotte-Marquez, J., Panisset, M., et al. (2009). Mild cognitive impairment in rapid eye movement sleep behavior disorder and Parkinson's disease. *Annals of Neurology, 66*(1), 39–47.

Gaig, C., Graus, F., Compta, Y., Hogl, B., Bataller, L., Bruggemann, N., et al. (2017). Clinical manifestations of the anti-IgLON5 disease. *Neurology, 88*(18), 1736–1743.

Gaig, C., Iranzo, A., Pujol, M., Perez, H., & Santamaria, J. (2017). Periodic limb movements during sleep mimicking REM sleep behavior disorder: A new form of periodic limb movement disorder. *Sleep, 40*(3). https://doi.org/10.1093/sleep/zsw063.

Gan-Or, Z., Mirelman, A., Postuma, R. B., Arnulf, I., Bar-Shira, A., Dauvilliers, Y., et al. (2015). GBA mutations are associated with rapid eye movement sleep behavior disorder. *Annals of Clinical and Translational Neurology, 2*(9), 941–945.

Gan-Or, Z., Ruskey, J. A., Spiegelman, D., Arnulf, I., Dauvilliers, Y., Hogl, B., et al. (2017). Heterozygous PINK1 p.G411S in rapid eye movement sleep behaviour disorder. *Brain: A Journal of Neurology, 140*(6), e32.

Garcia-Lorenzo, D., Longo-Dos Santos, C., Ewenczyk, C., Leu-Semenescu, S., Gallea, C., Quattrocchi, G., et al. (2013). The coeruleus/subcoeruleus complex in rapid eye movement sleep behaviour disorders in Parkinson's disease. *Brain: A Journal of Neurology, 136*(Pt 7), 2120–2129.

Haba-Rubio, J., Frauscher, B., Marques-Vidal, P., Toriel, J., Tobback, N., Andries, D., et al. (2017). Prevalence and determinants of REM sleep behavior disorder in the general population. *Sleep*.

Holtbernd, F., Gagnon, J. F., Postuma, R. B., Ma, Y., Tang, C. C., Feigin, A., et al. (2014). Abnormal metabolic network activity in REM sleep behavior disorder. *Neurology, 82*(7), 620–627.

Iranzo, A., & Santamaria, J. (2005). Severe obstructive sleep apnea/hypopnea mimicking REM sleep behavior disorder. *Sleep, 28*(2), 203–206.

Iranzo, A., Fernandez-Arcos, A., Tolosa, E., Serradell, M., Molinuevo, J. L., Valldeoriola, F., et al. (2014). Neurodegenerative disorder risk in idiopathic REM sleep behavior disorder: Study in 174 patients. *PLoS One, 9*(2), e89741.

Iranzo, A., Isetta, V., Molinuevo, J. L., Serradell, M., Navajas, D., Farre, R., et al. (2010). Electroencephalographic slowing heralds mild cognitive impairment in idiopathic REM sleep behavior disorder. *Sleep Medicine, 11*(6), 534–539.

Iranzo, A., Lomena, F., Stockner, H., Valldeoriola, F., Vilaseca, I., Salamero, M., et al. (2010). Decreased striatal dopamine transporter uptake and substantia nigra hyperechogenicity as risk markers of synucleinopathy in patients with idiopathic rapid-eye-movement sleep behaviour disorder: A prospective study [corrected]. *The Lancet Neurology, 9*(11), 1070–1077.

Iranzo, A., Santamaria, J., Valldeoriola, F., Serradell, M., Salamero, M., Gaig, C., et al. (2017). Dopamine transporter imaging deficit predicts early transition to synucleinopathy in idiopathic rapid eye movement sleep behavior disorder. *Annals of Neurology, 82*(3), 419–428.

Iranzo, A., Stockner, H., Serradell, M., Seppi, K., Valldeoriola, F., Frauscher, B., et al. (2014). Five-year follow-up of substantia nigra echogenicity in idiopathic REM sleep behavior disorder. *Movement Disorders: Official Journal of the Movement Disorder Society, 29*(14), 1774–1780.

Iranzo, A., Valldeoriola, F., Lomena, F., Molinuevo, J. L., Serradell, M., Salamero, M., et al. (2011). Serial dopamine transporter imaging of nigrostriatal function in patients with idiopathic rapid-eye-movement sleep behaviour disorder: A prospective study. *The Lancet Neurology, 10*(9), 797–805.

Kang, S. H., Yoon, I. Y., Lee, S. D., Han, J. W., Kim, T. H., & Kim, K. W. (2013). REM sleep behavior disorder in the Korean elderly population: Prevalence and clinical characteristics. *Sleep, 36*(8), 1147–1152.

Kim, K. T., Motamedi, G. K., & Cho, Y. W. (2017). Quality of life in patients with an idiopathic rapid eye movement sleep behaviour disorder in Korea. *Journal of Sleep Research, 26*(4), 422−427.

Kim, Y. E., Yang, H. J., Yun, J. Y., Kim, H. J., Lee, J. Y., & Jeon, B. S. (2014). REM sleep behavior disorder in Parkinson disease: Association with abnormal ocular motor findings. *Parkinsonism & Related Disorders, 20*(4), 444−446.

Kunz, D., & Mahlberg, R. (2010). A two-part, double-blind, placebo-controlled trial of exogenous melatonin in REM sleep behaviour disorder. *Journal of Sleep Research, 19*(4), 591−596.

Lam, S. P., Wong, C. C., Li, S. X., Zhang, J. H., Chan, J. W., Zhou, J. Y., et al. (2016). Caring burden of REM sleep behavior disorder - spouses' health and marital relationship. *Sleep Medicine, 24*, 40−43.

Lapierre, O., & Montplaisir, J. (1992). Polysomnographic features of REM sleep behavior disorder: Development of a scoring method. *Neurology, 42*(7), 1371−1374.

Mahlknecht, P., Iranzo, A., Hogl, B., Frauscher, B., Muller, C., Santamaria, J., et al. (2015). Olfactory dysfunction predicts early transition to a Lewy body disease in idiopathic RBD. *Neurology.*

Mahlknecht, P., Seppi, K., Frauscher, B., Kiechl, S., Willeit, J., Stockner, H., et al. (2015). Probable RBD and association with neurodegenerative disease markers: A population-based study. *Movement Disorders: Official Journal of the Movement Disorder Society, 30*(10), 1417−1421.

Mahowald, M. W., Bundlie, S. R., Hurwitz, T. D., & Schenck, C. H. (1990). Sleep violence–forensic science implications: Polygraphic and video documentation. *Journal of Forensic Sciences, 35*(2), 413−432.

Ma, C., Pavlova, M., Liu, Y., Liu, Y., Huangfu, C., Wu, S., et al. (2017). Probable REM sleep behavior disorder and risk of stroke: A prospective study. *Neurology, 88*(19), 1849−1855.

Ma, J. F., Qiao, Y., Gao, X., Liang, L., Liu, X. L., Li, D. H., et al. (2017). A community-based study of risk factors for probable rapid eye movement sleep behavior disorder. *Sleep Medicine, 30*, 71−76.

Mayer, G., Bitterlich, M., Kuwert, T., Ritt, P., & Stefan, H. (2015). Ictal SPECT in patients with rapid eye movement sleep behaviour disorder. *Brain: A Journal of Neurology, 138*(Pt 5), 1263−1270.

McCarter, S. J., St Louis, E. K., Duwell, E. J., Timm, P. C., Sandness, D. J., Boeve, B. F., et al. (2014). Diagnostic thresholds for quantitative REM sleep phasic burst duration, phasic and tonic muscle activity, and REM atonia index in REM sleep behavior disorder with and without comorbid obstructive sleep apnea. *Sleep, 37*(10), 1649−1662.

Montplaisir, J., Gagnon, J. F., Fantini, M. L., Postuma, R. B., Dauvilliers, Y., Desautels, A., et al. (2010). Polysomnographic diagnosis of idiopathic REM sleep behavior disorder. *Movement Disorders: Official Journal of the Movement Disorder Society, 25*(13), 2044−2051.

Nomura, T., Inoue, Y., Hogl, B., Uemura, Y., Kitayama, M., Abe, T., et al. (2010). Relationship between (123)I-MIBG scintigrams and REM sleep behavior disorder in Parkinson's disease. *Parkinsonism & Related Disorders, 16*(10), 683−685.

Olson, E. J., Boeve, B. F., & Silber, M. H. (2000). Rapid eye movement sleep behaviour disorder: Demographic, clinical and laboratory findings in 93 cases. *Brain: A Journal of Neurology, 123*(Pt 2), 331−339.

Oudiette, D., De Cock, V. C., Lavault, S., Leu, S., Vidailhet, M., & Arnulf, I. (2009). Nonviolent elaborate behaviors may also occur in REM sleep behavior disorder. *Neurology, 72*(6), 551−557.

Pont-Sunyer, C., Iranzo, A., Gaig, C., Fernandez-Arcos, A., Vilas, D., Valldeoriola, F., et al. (2015). Sleep disorders in parkinsonian and nonparkinsonian LRRK2 mutation carriers. *PLoS One, 10*(7), e0132368.

Postuma, R. B., Gagnon, J. F., Rompre, S., & Montplaisir, J. Y. (2010). Severity of REM atonia loss in idiopathic REM sleep behavior disorder predicts Parkinson disease. *Neurology, 74*(3), 239−244.

Postuma, R. B., Gagnon, J. F., Tuineaig, M., Bertrand, J. A., Latreille, V., Desjardins, C., et al. (2013). Antidepressants and REM sleep behavior disorder: Isolated side effect or neurodegenerative signal? *Sleep, 36*(11), 1579−1585.

Postuma, R. B., Gagnon, J. F., Vendette, M., Charland, K., & Montplaisir, J. (2008). REM sleep behaviour disorder in Parkinson's disease is associated with specific motor features. *Journal of Neurology, Neurosurgery & Psychiatry, 79*(10), 1117−1121.

Postuma, R. B., Gagnon, J. F., Vendette, M., Fantini, M. L., Massicotte-Marquez, J., & Montplaisir, J. (2009). Quantifying the risk of neurodegenerative disease in idiopathic REM sleep behavior disorder. *Neurology, 72*(15), 1296−1300.

Postuma, R. B., Gagnon, J. F., Vendette, M., & Montplaisir, J. Y. (2009a). Idiopathic REM sleep behavior disorder in the transition to degenerative disease. *Movement Disorders: Official Journal of the Movement Disorder Society, 24*(15), 2225−2232.

Postuma, R. B., Gagnon, J. F., Vendette, M., & Montplaisir, J. Y. (2009b). Markers of neurodegeneration in idiopathic rapid eye movement sleep behaviour disorder and Parkinson's disease. *Brain: A Journal of Neurology, 132*(Pt 12), 3298−3307.

Postuma, R. B., Iranzo, A., Hogl, B., Arnulf, I., Ferini-Strambi, L., Manni, R., et al. (2015). Risk factors for neurodegeneration in idiopathic rapid eye movement sleep behavior disorder: A multicenter study. *Annals of Neurology, 77*(5), 830−839.

Postuma, R. B., Iranzo, A., Hu, M., Hogl, B., Boeve, B. F., Manni, R., et al. (2019). Risk and predictors of dementia and parkinsonism in idiopathic REM sleep behaviour disorder: A multicentre study. *Brain: A Journal of Neurology, 142*(3), 744−759.

Postuma, R. B., Lang, A. E., Massicotte-Marquez, J., & Montplaisir, J. (2006). Potential early markers of Parkinson disease in idiopathic REM sleep behavior disorder. *Neurology, 66*(6), 845−851.

Postuma, R. B., Montplaisir, J. Y., Pelletier, A., Dauvilliers, Y., Oertel, W., Iranzo, A., et al. (2012). Environmental risk factors for REM sleep behavior disorder: A multicenter case-control study. *Neurology, 79*(5), 428−434.

Pujol, M., Pujol, J., Alonso, T., Fuentes, A., Pallerola, M., Freixenet, J., et al. (2017). Idiopathic REM sleep behavior disorder in the elderly Spanish community: A primary care center study with a two-stage design using video-polysomnography. *Sleep Medicine, 40*, 116−121.

Sabater, L., Gaig, C., Gelpi, E., Bataller, L., Lewerenz, J., Torres-Vega, E., et al. (2014). A novel non-rapid-eye movement and rapid-eye-movement parasomnia with sleep breathing disorder associated with antibodies to IgLON5: A case series, characterisation of the antigen, and post-mortem study. *The Lancet Neurology, 13*(6), 575−586.

Sixel-Doring, F., Schweitzer, M., Mollenhauer, B., & Trenkwalder, C. (2009). Polysomnographic findings, video-based sleep analysis and sleep perception in progressive supranuclear palsy. *Sleep Medicine, 10*(4), 407−415.

St Louis, E. K., Boeve, A. R., & Boeve, B. F. (2017). REM sleep behavior disorder in Parkinson's disease and other synucleinopathies. *Movement Disorders: Official Journal of the Movement Disorder Society, 32*(5), 645–658.

Stefani, A., Gabelia, D., Hogl, B., Mitterling, T., Mahlknecht, P., Stockner, H., et al. (2015). Long-term follow-up investigation of isolated rapid eye movement sleep without atonia without rapid eye movement sleep behavior disorder: A pilot study. *Journal of Clinical Sleep Medicine: Official Publication of the American Academy of Sleep Medicine, 11*(11), 1273–1279.

Stiasny-Kolster, K., Mayer, G., Schafer, S., Moller, J. C., Heinzel-Gutenbrunner, M., & Oertel, W. H. (2007). The REM sleep behavior disorder screening questionnaire–a new diagnostic instrument. *Movement Disorders: Official Journal of the Movement Disorder Society, 22*(16), 2386–2393.

Teman, P. T., Tippmann-Peikert, M., Silber, M. H., Slocumb, N. L., & Auger, R. R. (2009). Idiopathic rapid-eye-movement sleep disorder: Associations with antidepressants, psychiatric diagnoses, and other factors, in relation to age of onset. *Sleep Medicine, 10*(1), 60–65.

Uribe-San Martin, R., Venegas Francke, P., Lopez Illanes, F., Jones Gazmuri, A., Salazar Rivera, J., Godoy Fernndez, J., et al. (2013). Plasma urate in REM sleep behavior disorder. *Movement Disorders: Official Journal of the Movement Disorder Society, 28*(8), 1150–1151.

Wong, J. C., Li, J., Pavlova, M., Chen, S., Wu, A., Wu, S., et al. (2016). Risk factors for probable REM sleep behavior disorder: A community-based study. *Neurology, 86*(14), 1306–1312.

Zhang, J., Lam, S. P., Ho, C. K., Li, A. M., Tsoh, J., Mok, V., et al. (2008). Diagnosis of REM sleep behavior disorder by video-polysomnographic study: Is one night enough? *Sleep, 31*(8), 1179–1185.

Restless legs syndrome and periodic limb movements

Illustrative case

A 56-year-old woman with Parkinson's disease (PD) presents for follow-up. She has moderate PD and is being treated with levodopa 200 mg three times a day along with pramipexole 1 mg three times a day. Her last dose of dopaminergic medication is taken at around 6:00 p.m. She feels her motor symptoms are generally well controlled on this regimen, though sometimes she has stiffness when her dose of PD medications wears off. However, she complains of discomfort in her legs that has been keeping her up at night. This began a few years ago but has now gotten to the point where it is much more bothersome and disruptive to her sleep. She reports that in the evening, always around 9:30 p.m. when she lies down in bed, she gets a feeling in her legs that she describes as "like ants crawling all over them." She will get out of bed and walk around her bedroom, and the feeling goes away. However, when she lies back down, the feeling recurs. When these symptoms started to occur, they were only a few times a month and mild but more recently they are much more severe, occurring almost nightly and on some nights can keep her up for several hours.

Overview
Definition

Restless legs syndrome (RLS) and periodic limb movement disorder (PLMD) are both sleep-related movement disorders and are considered here together, although they are distinct disorders.

RLS is also known as Willis-Ekbom disease. According to the international classification of sleep disorders, version 3 (ICSD III) criteria (American Academy of Sleep Medicine, 2014), its diagnosis requires "an urge to move the legs, usually accompanied by uncomfortable and unpleasant sensations in the legs." Symptoms must begin or worsen during times of relative inactivity, must at least be partially relieved by movement, and must cause distress and/or impairment of function.

The International Restless Legs Syndrome Study Group consensus diagnostic criteria (Allen et al., 2014) require all of the following to be present for RLS diagnosis:

1. "An urge to move the legs usually but not always accompanied by, or felt to be caused by, uncomfortable and unpleasant sensations in the legs
2. The urge to move the legs and any accompanying unpleasant sensations begin or worsen during periods of rest or inactivity such as lying down or sitting
3. The urge to move the legs and any accompanying unpleasant sensations are partially or totally relieved by movement, such as walking or stretching, at least as long as the activity continues.
4. The urge to move the legs and any accompanying unpleasant sensations during rest or inactivity only occur or are worse in the evening or night than during the day.
5. The occurrence of the above features is not solely accounted for as symptoms primary to another medical or a behavioral condition (e.g., myalgia, venous stasis, leg edema, arthritis, leg cramps, positional discomfort, habitual foot tapping)"

The diagnosis of RLS in PD is challenging as compared to primary (idiopathic) RLS (RLS occurring in an individual without comorbid PD or other neurologic disorder) (Hogl & Stefani, 2017). Nonspecific leg restlessness is common in PD, but may not necessarily otherwise meet the criteria for RLS as defined for the general population.

RLS symptom frequency varies from one patient to another and within-subject. Some patients have nightly symptoms, whereas others experience infrequent symptoms that are very context-specific.

PLMD is also a sleep-related movement disorder. It is marked by the occurrence of periodic limb movements during sleep (PLMS) that must be associated with clinically significant sleep disturbance or impairment of functioning (American Academy of Sleep Medicine, 2014). The frequency of PLMS that is considered abnormal is >5/hour in children and >15/hour in adults. PLMS are obviously required for a diagnosis of PLMD, but occurrence of PLMS also may occur in isolation, in the absence of clinically significant sleep disturbance or impairment in functioning. In addition, PLMs are also seen in other disorders. To the latter point, PLMs are often seen in patients with RLS; PLMs occurring in a patient with RLS cannot be separately diagnosed as PLMD (Hogl & Stefani, 2017). The International Classification of Sleep Disorders—version 3 specifically states, in this regard, that "the diagnosis of RLS takes precedence over that of PLMD when potentially sleep-disrupting PLMS occur in the context of RLS" (American Academy of Sleep Medicine, 2014).

Validated objective measures of RLS in PD are lacking, but some data indicate that the suggested immobilization test may be of utility for RLS diagnosis in PD, at least in the research setting. The original validated version of this test (Michaud, Lavigne, Desautels, Poirier, & Montplaisir, 2002) was administered at

9:00 p.m., and consisted of the subject reclining with legs outstretched, for 60 minutes and told to resist voluntary movement as long as is possible. Subject discomfort was measured with a visual analogue scale, and leg movements were quantified with surface EMG applied to the tibialis anterior muscle. In a study applying the suggested immobilization test to 25 PD patients with a clinical diagnosis of RLS and 25 age- and gender-matched PD patients without RLS, severity of leg discomfort was measured with a visual analogue scale with possible responses ranging from ranging from 0 (no discomfort) to 100 (extreme discomfort). This was assessed every 10 minutes during the 1-hour immobilization test that was started at 8:00 p.m. A mean leg discomfort score cutoff of 11 had a sensitivity of 91% and specificity of 72% for RLS diagnosis (De Cock et al., 2012).

Epidemiology

The study of the epidemiology of RLS in PD is made challenging by the common occurrence of leg restlessness in PD that does not meet criteria for RLS. A study by Gjerstad et al. that considered leg restlessness versus RLS diagnosis based on diagnostic criteria from the general population illustrates this (Gjerstad, Tysnes, & Larsen, 2011). That study investigated leg restlessness in 200 drug-naïve PD patients and 173 age- and gender-matched controls (Gjerstad et al., 2011). Leg restlessness was ascertained by structured interview, and a diagnosis if RLS was made according to diagnostic criteria (Allen et al., 2003). 40% of the PD patients reported leg restlessness compared to 18% of controls. Despite the 40% prevalence of leg restlessness in the cohort, only 15% of the PD cohort met diagnostic criteria for RLS (40% of those with leg restlessness). RLS mimics identified in the PD group included neuropathy, radiculopathy, arthritis, and nonspecific pain/sensory symptoms. The relative risk for RLS in the PD cohort was 1.76, whereas the relative risk for leg motor restlessness was 2.84. Similarly, in another study investigating leg restlessness and RLS in 436 PD patients and 401 age- and gender- matched controls (Suzuki et al., 2017), the prevalence of RLS was not different in the PD versus non-PD group (3.4% vs. 2.7%). In contrast, leg motor restlessness was significantly more common in the PD group compared to the non-PD group (12.8% vs. 4.5%).

A few subsequent studies did find that RLS is more common in PD than in the general population (Calzetti, Angelini, Negrotti, Marchesi, & Goldoni, 2014) and in PD compared to other neurodegenerative parkinsonian disorders (Bhalsing, Suresh, Muthane, & Pal, 2013). However again, in interpreting these data, the challenges of diagnosing RLS in PD must be kept in mind.

The reported RLS prevalence in PD ranges from 3% to 21.3% (Azmin et al., 2013; Loo & Tan, 2008; Rana et al., 2013; Verbaan, van Rooden, van Hilten, & Rijsman, 2010). Reported prevalence of RLS diagnosed based on structured interview is substantially lower than that reported in studies that ascertained RLS based on questionnaire responses, likely reflecting the inability of questionnaires to consistently distinguish between RLS and leg motor restlessness. For example, as compared to the 3.4% prevalence of RLS found based on structured interview

(Suzuki et al., 2017), in a study of 577 PD patients who responded to a questionnaire on RLS, RLS occurred in 20.3% of cases (Ylikoski, Martikainen, & Partinen, 2015). Whether RLS in PD relates to specific demographics or greater disease severity in PD is not clear; there are conflicting results as to whether RLS is more common in male PD patients compared to female PD patients, in those with younger versus older age of onset, and in relation to disease stage (Azmin et al., 2013; Bhalsing et al., 2013). In those with older age of PD onset, RLS may develop earlier in the disease course (in relation to onset of PD symptoms/diagnosis) compared to younger patients (Nomura, Inoue, & Nakashima, 2009).

As for RLS preceding the diagnosis of PD, one study in a large epidemiologic cohort indicated that RLS may be an early manifestation of PD; it is thus a prodromal feature but is not seen as a risk factor for PD per se (Wong, Li, Schwarzschild, Ascherio, & Gao, 2014).

There are few data on the prevalence of PLMD in PD, and on the implications of PLMS in PD. Some studies report an association between presence of PLMS and RLS in PD (Loo & Tan, 2008) whereas this was not demonstrated in other studies (Prudon, Duncan, Khoo, Yarnall, & Anderson, 2014); indeed, one study found PLMS to be more common in non-PD patients with RLS compared to PD patients with RLS On the other hand, PD patients with RLS did not have significantly more PLMS compared to PD patients without RLS (De Cock et al., 2012).

Etiology and differential diagnosis

Pathophysiologically, RLS is seen as a dopamine-deficiency disorder, similar to PD. In that sense, their co-occurrence is not surprising. However, in primary RLS, striatal dopaminergic denervation is not seen, at least not to the degree it is seen in PD (Linke et al., 2004). Of interest, and in contrast, PD is seen as a disorder of iron excess (excess deposition of iron in the brain) whereas in primary RLS, a relative iron deficiency is seen pathologically, and this has clinical correlates (iron deficiency is an etiology of or contributors to RLS). These differences are reflected in sonographic findings in the substantia nigra in these two patient populations: substantia nigra hyperechogenicity is seen in PD (Berg, Merz, Reiners, Naumann, & Becker, 2005) whereas in RLS patients (without PD), the substantia nigra is hypoechoic (Schmidauer et al., 2005). As for substantia nigra transcranial doppler ultrasonography findings in PD patients with RLS, one study compared TCD findings in 26 PD patients with RLS to 37 PD patients without RLS and 40 primary RLS cases (Kwon et al., 2010). Significant hyperechogenicity in the substantia nigra was seen in both PD groups compared to the primary RLS group and the RLS group did have relative hypoechogenicity. The authors interpreted their results to possibly mean that RLS pathophysiology in PD is different from RLS pathophysiology in the general population. Similar findings were seen in another study of PD + RLS compared to primary RLS (Ryu, Lee, & Baik, 2011). Clearly, additional work is needed to clarify the role of iron in pathophysiology of RLS in general and as it relates to PD.

Although a heritability of RLS in PD is not confirmed, in the general population with primary RLS, a family history of RLS is common. Regarding genetic contributions to RLS pathophysiology, in a study of 258 RLS patients compared to 235 without RLS, a lower prevalence of the longest size variant (allele 2) of the complex microsatellite repeat Rep1 within the SNCA gene was found in the RLS group (Lahut et al., 2014). This is in contrast to PD, where this allele 2 of the Rep1 gene is associated with increased risk of PD. The role of alpha-synuclein in RLS pathophysiology, and its relationship to dopaminergic abnormalities seen in these two disorders is not known but warrants further study.

As mentioned earlier, several factors complicate the diagnosis of RLS in PD, and several mimics of RLS require consideration in PD (Table 7.1) (Hening, Allen, Washburn, Lesage, & Earley, 2009; Hogl & Stefani, 2017). Most saliently is that leg restlessness in PD is common (Gjerstad et al., 2011; Rajabally & Martey, 2013; Suzuki et al., 2012) but there are often not the historical features present that support the diagnosis of RLS based on core criteria. For example, PD patients with a clear history of leg restlessness may not have a history consistent with worsening in the evening/night or relief with activity (Gjerstad et al., 2011) (see epidemiology section).

An urge to move the legs and unpleasant sensations in the legs may be a manifestation of wearing off of dopaminergic medications (Peralta et al., 2005). When these sensations/urges are strictly linked to PD medication wearing off and improve with medication intake, a diagnosis of RLS cannot be made.

In the non-PD population, RLS may be a manifestation of other comorbidities (Table 7.1). These should be considered in a PD patient with symptoms of RLS, where appropriate.

Otherwise, there are several RLS mimics and differential diagnoses to be considered (Table 7.2).

Table 7.1 Causes of RLS (secondary RLS).

Disorder	Comment
Anemia	May account, in part, for increased RLS risk seen in pregnancy. Acute RLS may follow blood donation
Spinal anesthesia	RLS following spinal anesthesia may be transient
Neuropathy	RLS may be seen in patients with neuropathies of various etiologies. However, neuropathic symptoms may also be a mimic of RLS. This distinction is made based on the history provided
Thyroid disorders	RLS is rarely a manifestation of hypothyroidism
Medications	Selective serotonin reuptake inhibitors and serotonin norepinephrine reuptake inhibitors may cause or exacerbate RLS

Table 7.2 Conditions to be considered in the differential diagnosis of RLS.

Venous stasis
Leg edema
Arthritis/other musculoskeletal problems
Leg cramps
Peripheral nervous system disorder (neuropathy/radiculopathy)
Radiculopathy
Habitual foot tapping/leg shaking
Dystonia
Akathisia
Dyskinesias

Consequences and complications

PD patients with RLS report worse quality of life as compared to those without RLS (Covassin et al., 2012; Ylikoski et al., 2015). In addition, RLS in PD has been associated with worse subjective sleep quality (Suzuki et al., 2017; Ylikoski et al., 2015) and daytime sleepiness (Suzuki et al., 2017; Ylikoski et al., 2015). RLS in PD may cause or contribute to sleep onset insomnia (see Chapter 1) and sleep maintenance insomnia (see Chapter 2) (Yu et al., 2013). Objectively, one study found that RLS in PD is associated with reduced sleep efficiency (Loo & Tan, 2008) though this was not replicated in a subsequent study (Covassin et al., 2012). PLMS in PD are also associated with worse subjective sleep quality (Covassin et al., 2012). RLS in PD is often comorbid with other sleep disorders.

RLS in PD is associated with several nonmotor symptoms of PD. RLS severity in PD is associated with cognitive dysfunction, as well as symptoms of depression and psychosis (Neikrug et al., 2013; Verbaan et al., 2010). It is also associated with excessive daytime sleepiness (see Chapter 12). In addition, PD patients with RLS are more likely to have symptoms of autonomic dysfunction (Chung et al., 2013; Kurtis, Rodriguez-Blazquez, Martinez-Martin, & ELEP Group, 2013; Tijero et al., 2011).

To what degree RLS causes these nonmotor features or if they are just manifestations of underlying neurodegeneration affecting pathways relevant to all of them is not clear. It may be a combination of both the latter explanations.

Although, in one study, evidence of peripheral neuropathy and serum vitamin B12 levels were not found to be significantly different in PD patients with RLS compared to those without (Rajabally & Martey, 2013), data in this regard are limited, and these should nevertheless be considered in evaluating the PD patient with RLS, to identify potential treatable causes.

In the non-PD population, PLMD has been associated with increased risk of cardiovascular disease. There are few data on this in the PD population.

Management

Given that iron deficiency can cause or worsen RLS, all patients should be screened with ferritin level at diagnosis and periodically thereafter. Oral iron supplementation is indicated when serum ferritin ≤ 75 µg/L (Winkelman et al., 2016). In PD patients, iron supplementation may exacerbate constipation and proactive management of that, either with prescription of stool softeners, and/or consideration of iron formulations less likely to cause constipation (such as ferrous gluconate) may be necessary. The effects that oral iron supplementation could have on levodopa absorption have to be kept in mind as well (intake of iron supplements should be timed so as not to be taken too close to levodopa doses).

A nonpharmacologic option with moderate level of evidence that may be useful in some patients include pneumatic compression (Winkelman et al., 2016), applied in the evening before typical time of RLS symptom onset. The utility of this in the PD population with RLS is unknown.

As for pharmacotherapy, the highest level of evidence for efficacy in treating RLS in the general population is for pramipexole, rotigotine, and gabapentin enacarbil (Garcia-Borreguero et al., 2016; Winkelman et al., 2016). This is followed by ropinirole and then levodopa. Other treatments with less evidence include gabapentin and pregabalin. In managing RLS, augmentation should be monitored for regularly. Augmentation is a phenomenon whereby RLS symptoms start to worsen, occurring earlier in the day. With the risk of augmentation in mind, in the non-PD population, it has been suggested that gabapentin enacarbil be the first-line therapy for treatment of RLS, to minimize risk of augmentation (Garcia-Borreguero et al., 2016). Dopamine agonists and especially levodopa carry higher risk of augmentation. In cases refractory to other options, and especially if augmentation is present, opioids may be required to control symptoms.

There are few data to guide treatment of RLS specifically in the PD population. In PD, rationale use of dopaminergic medications to treat both RLS and other manifestations of PD is recommended. Other drug classes such as gabapentin/gabapentin enacarbil have not been well studied specifically in the PD population with RLS but should be considered where necessary, especially in PD patients who do not tolerate agonists and/or develop augmentation.

An important consideration in the management of RLS in PD relates to the possible emergence of RLS with reductions in dopaminergic medications. This is particularly important to keep in mind if patients undergo advanced surgical therapies such as deep brain stimulation surgery (DBS). Although some patients with PD have an improvement in their RLS symptoms following DBS (Chahine, Ahmed, & Sun, 2011; Driver-Dunckley et al., 2006), in other patients, an emergence of RLS occurs postoperatively (Kedia, Moro, Tagliati, Lang, & Kumar, 2004). The latter may relate to reductions in doses of dopaminergic medication that may occur in some patients following DBS.

As mentioned, PLMs do not necessarily need to be treated unless they lead to arousals/sleep disturbance. Ropinirole has the strongest level of evidence for efficacy for symptomatic PLMs in the general population (Winkelman et al., 2016).

Illustrative case in context

The patient depicted in the case has PD and a history consistent with RLS. Although symptoms have been increasing in frequency and severity, there is no indication that they are occurring earlier in the day, making augmentation less of a concern at this time. As the symptoms sound very bothersome to her and are impacting her sleep, treatment is indicated. As a first step, ferritin level should be checked and oral iron supplementation initiated. A stool softener is ideally started along with the iron, and the doses of iron supplementation should be timed so that they are not too close to levodopa doses (since oral iron supplements can interfere with levodopa absorption). If this is insufficient to help her symptoms, a bedtime dose of gabapentin enacarbil would be a good first step. If cost is a concern, it is likely gabapentin enacarbil would be effective too, despite limited evidence. If this is insufficient to control her symptoms, and especially if/when nighttime motor problems are an issue, switching her immediate release daytime pramipexole to a long-acting bedtime dose of pramipexole would be a good next step.

References

Allen, R. P., Picchietti, D. L., Garcia-Borreguero, D., Ondo, W. G., Walters, A. S., Winkelman, J. W., et al. (2014). Restless legs syndrome/Willis-Ekbom disease diagnostic criteria: Updated international restless legs syndrome study group (IRLSSG) consensus criteria–history, rationale, description, and significance. *Sleep Medicine, 15*(8), 860–873.

Allen, R. P., Picchietti, D., Hening, W. A., Trenkwalder, C., Walters, A. S., Montplaisi, J., et al. (2003). Restless legs syndrome: Diagnostic criteria, special considerations, and epidemiology. A report from the restless legs syndrome diagnosis and epidemiology workshop at the National Institutes of Health. *Sleep Medicine, 4*(2), 101–119.

American Academy of Sleep Medicine. (2014). *International classification of sleep disorders* (3rd ed.). Darien, IL: American Academy of Sleep Medicine.

Azmin, S., Khairul Anuar, A. M., Nafisah, W. Y., Tan, H. J., Raymond, A. A., Hanita, O., et al. (2013). Restless legs syndrome and its associated risk factors in Parkinson's disease. *Parkinson's Disease, 2013*, 535613.

Berg, D., Merz, B., Reiners, K., Naumann, M., & Becker, G. (2005). Five-year follow-up study of hyperechogenicity of the substantia nigra in Parkinson's disease. *Movement Disorders: Official Journal of the Movement Disorder Society, 20*(3), 383–385.

Bhalsing, K., Suresh, K., Muthane, U. B., & Pal, P. K. (2013). Prevalence and profile of restless legs syndrome in Parkinson's disease and other neurodegenerative disorders: A case-control study. *Parkinsonism & Related Disorders, 19*(4), 426–430.

Calzetti, S., Angelini, M., Negrotti, A., Marchesi, E., & Goldoni, M. (2014). A long-term prospective follow-up study of incident RLS in the course of chronic DAergic therapy in newly diagnosed untreated patients with Parkinson's disease. *Journal of Neural Transmission, 121*(5), 499−506.

Chahine, L. M., Ahmed, A., & Sun, Z. (2011). Effects of STN DBS for Parkinson's disease on restless legs syndrome and other sleep-related measures. *Parkinsonism & Related Disorders, 17*(3), 208−211.

Chung, S., Bohnen, N. I., Albin, R. L., Frey, K. A., Muller, M. L., & Chervin, R. D. (2013). Insomnia and sleepiness in Parkinson disease: Associations with symptoms and comorbidities. *Journal of Clinical Sleep Medicine: Official Publication of the American Academy of Sleep Medicine, 9*(11), 1131−1137.

Covassin, N., Neikrug, A. B., Liu, L., Corey-Bloom, J., Loredo, J. S., Palmer, B. W., et al. (2012). Clinical correlates of periodic limb movements in sleep in Parkinson's disease. *Journal of the Neurological Sciences, 316*(1−2), 131−136.

De Cock, V. C., Bayard, S., Yu, H., Grini, M., Carlander, B., Postuma, R., et al. (2012). Suggested immobilization test for diagnosis of restless legs syndrome in Parkinson's disease. *Movement Disorders: Official Journal of the Movement Disorder Society, 27*(6), 743−749.

Driver-Dunckley, E., Evidente, V. G., Adler, C. H., Hillman, R., Hernandez, J., Fletcher, G., et al. (2006). Restless legs syndrome in Parkinson's disease patients may improve with subthalamic stimulation. *Movement Disorders: Official Journal of the Movement Disorder Society, 21*(8), 1287−1289.

Garcia-Borreguero, D., Silber, M. H., Winkelman, J. W., Hogl, B., Bainbridge, J., Buchfuhrer, M., et al. (2016). Guidelines for the first-line treatment of restless legs syndrome/Willis-Ekbom disease, prevention and treatment of dopaminergic augmentation: A combined task force of the IRLSSG, EURLSSG, and the RLS-foundation. *Sleep Medicine, 21*, 1−11.

Gjerstad, M. D., Tysnes, O. B., & Larsen, J. P. (2011). Increased risk of leg motor restlessness but not RLS in early Parkinson disease. *Neurology, 77*(22), 1941−1946.

Hening, W. A., Allen, R. P., Washburn, M., Lesage, S. R., & Earley, C. J. (2009). The four diagnostic criteria for Restless Legs Syndrome are unable to exclude confounding conditions ("mimics"). *Sleep Medicine, 10*(9), 976−981.

Hogl, B., & Stefani, A. (2017). Restless legs syndrome and periodic leg movements in patients with movement disorders: Specific considerations. *Movement Disorders: Official Journal of the Movement Disorder Society, 32*(5), 669−681.

Kedia, S., Moro, E., Tagliati, M., Lang, A. E., & Kumar, R. (2004). Emergence of restless legs syndrome during subthalamic stimulation for Parkinson disease. *Neurology, 63*(12), 2410−2412.

Kurtis, M. M., Rodriguez-Blazquez, C., Martinez-Martin, P., & ELEP Group. (2013). Relationship between sleep disorders and other non-motor symptoms in Parkinson's disease. *Parkinsonism & Related Disorders, 19*(12), 1152−1155.

Kwon, D. Y., Seo, W. K., Yoon, H. K., Park, M. H., Koh, S. B., & Park, K. W. (2010). Transcranial brain sonography in Parkinson's disease with restless legs syndrome. *Movement Disorders: Official Journal of the Movement Disorder Society, 25*(10), 1373−1378.

Lahut, S., Vadasz, D., Depboylu, C., Ries, V., Krenzer, M., Stiasny-Kolster, K., et al. (2014). The PD-associated alpha-synuclein promoter Rep1 allele 2 shows diminished frequency in restless legs syndrome. *Neurogenetics, 15*(3), 189−192.

Linke, R., Eisensehr, I., Wetter, T. C., Gildehaus, F. J., Popperl, G., Trenkwalder, C., et al. (2004). Presynaptic dopaminergic function in patients with restless legs syndrome: Are there common features with early Parkinson's disease? *Movement Disorders: Official Journal of the Movement Disorder Society, 19*(10), 1158−1162.

Loo, H. V., & Tan, E. K. (2008). Case-control study of restless legs syndrome and quality of sleep in Parkinson's disease. *Journal of the Neurological Sciences, 266*(1−2), 145−149.

Michaud, M., Lavigne, G., Desautels, A., Poirier, G., & Montplaisir, J. (2002). Effects of immobility on sensory and motor symptoms of restless legs syndrome. *Movement Disorders: Official Journal of the Movement Disorder Society, 17*(1), 112−115.

Neikrug, A. B., Maglione, J. E., Liu, L., Natarajan, L., Avanzino, J. A., Corey-Bloom, J., et al. (2013). Effects of sleep disorders on the non-motor symptoms of Parkinson disease. *Journal of Clinical Sleep Medicine: Official Publication of the American Academy of Sleep Medicine, 9*(11), 1119−1129.

Nomura, T., Inoue, Y., & Nakashima, K. (2009). Pathogenetic heterogeneity of restless legs syndrome in Parkinson's disease. *Sleep and Biological Rhythms, 7*(1), 31−33.

Peralta, C. M., Wolf, E., Seppi, K., Wenning, G. K., Hogl, B., & Poewe, W. (2005). Restless legs in idiopathic Parkinson's disease [abstract]. *Movement Disorders, 20*(Suppl. 10), S108.

Prudon, B., Duncan, G. W., Khoo, T. K., Yarnall, A. J., & Anderson, K. N. (2014). Primary sleep disorder prevalence in patients with newly diagnosed Parkinson's disease. *Movement Disorders: Official Journal of the Movement Disorder Society, 29*(2), 259−262.

Rajabally, Y. A., & Martey, J. (2013). No association between neuropathy and restless legs in Parkinson's disease. *Acta Neurologica Scandinavica, 127*(3), 216−220.

Rana, A. Q., Siddiqui, I., Mosabbir, A., Athar, A., Syed, O., Jesudasan, M., et al. (2013). Association of pain, Parkinson's disease, and restless legs syndrome. *Journal of the Neurological Sciences, 327*(1−2), 32−34.

Ryu, J. H., Lee, M. S., & Baik, J. S. (2011). Sonographic abnormalities in idiopathic restless legs syndrome (RLS) and RLS in Parkinson's disease. *Parkinsonism & Related Disorders, 17*(3), 201−203.

Schmidauer, C., Sojer, M., Seppi, K., Stockner, H., Hogl, B., Biedermann, B., et al. (2005). Transcranial ultrasound shows nigral hypoechogenicity in restless legs syndrome. *Annals of Neurology, 58*(4), 630−634.

Suzuki, K., Miyamoto, M., Miyamoto, T., Tatsumoto, M., Watanabe, Y., Suzuki, S., et al. (2012). Nocturnal disturbances and restlessness in Parkinson's disease: Using the Japanese version of the Parkinson's disease sleep scale-2. *Journal of the Neurological Sciences, 318*(1−2), 76−81.

Suzuki, K., Okuma, Y., Uchiyama, T., Miyamoto, M., Sakakibara, R., Shimo, Y., et al. (2017). Characterizing restless legs syndrome and leg motor restlessness in patients with Parkinson's disease: A multicenter case-controlled study. *Parkinsonism & Related Disorders, 44*, 18−22.

Tijero, B., Somme, J., Gomez-Esteban, J. C., Berganzo, K., Adhikari, I., Lezcano, E., et al. (2011). Relationship between sleep and dysautonomic symptoms assessed by self-report scales. *Movement Disorders: Official Journal of the Movement Disorder Society, 26*(10), 1967−1968.

Verbaan, D., van Rooden, S. M., van Hilten, J. J., & Rijsman, R. M. (2010). Prevalence and clinical profile of restless legs syndrome in Parkinson's disease. *Movement Disorders: Official Journal of the Movement Disorder Society, 25*(13), 2142−2147.

Winkelman, J. W., Armstrong, M. J., Allen, R. P., Chaudhuri, K. R., Ondo, W., Trenkwalder, C., et al. (2016). Practice guideline summary: Treatment of restless legs syndrome in adults: Report of the guideline development, dissemination, and implementation subcommittee of the American Academy of Neurology. *Neurology, 87*(24), 2585–2593.

Wong, J. C., Li, Y., Schwarzschild, M. A., Ascherio, A., & Gao, X. (2014). Restless legs syndrome: An early clinical feature of Parkinson disease in men. *Sleep, 37*(2), 369–372.

Ylikoski, A., Martikainen, K., & Partinen, M. (2015). Parkinson's disease and restless legs syndrome. *European Neurology, 73*(3–4), 212–219.

Yu, S. Y., Sun, L., Liu, Z., Huang, X. Y., Zuo, L. J., Cao, C. J., et al. (2013). Sleep disorders in Parkinson's disease: Clinical features, iron metabolism and related mechanism. *PLoS One, 8*(12), e82924.

Sleep-related breathing disorders

Illustrative case

A 67-year-old man with Parkinson's disease of 8 years' duration reports increasing problems with daytime sleepiness. In recent years, he is dozing off more during the day. He feels like he sleeps a sufficient number of hours at night (at least 8) but still wakes up feeling unrefreshed. He denies any difficulty breathing during the night. His wife, on the other hand, reports that he snores loudly for most of the night and on several occasions has witnessed him to stop breathing for several seconds. These episodes are often followed by a sudden loud gasp. These are more likely to occur when he is sleeping on his back. His body mass index (BMI) is 31. He fills out an Epworth Sleepiness Scale and scores 17. He undergoes polysomnography (PSG) that shows an apnea-hypopnea index of 27.1, with an arousal index (number of microarousals per hour) of 22.1 and oxygen saturation nadir of 78%.

Overview

Definition

The International Classification of Sleep Disorders (American Academy of Sleep Medicine, 2014) recognizes four sleep-related breathing disorders: central sleep apnea syndromes, obstructive sleep apnea (OSA) syndromes, sleep-related hypoventilation disorders, and sleep-related hypoxemia disorders. Data on sleep-related hypoventilation disorders and sleep-related hypoxemia disorders in Parkinson's disease (PD) are limited but based on their occurrence and risk factors in the general population, these are likely relatively rare in PD and will not be further considered here.

The diagnosis of OSA is based on the apnea-hypopnea index (AHI) or the number of obstructive respiratory events (apneas, hypopneas, or respiratory effort—related arousals) that occur per hour. Obstructive respiratory events are defined by the American Academic of Sleep Medicine scoring guidelines (American Academy of Sleep Medicine, 2018) based on changes in airflow, along with arousals and/or oximetry. An AHI > 5 may be clinically relevant in some patient populations and >15 is considered diagnostic of OSA in adults, regardless of comorbidities.

Disorders of Sleep and Wakefulness in Parkinson's Disease. https://doi.org/10.1016/B978-0-323-67374-7.00008-0

Diagnosis of OSA is made based on history and PSG. Symptoms elicited on history may include snoring or gasping/choking episodes either reported by the patient and/or witnesses. However, snoring may not be reported in some PD patients with OSA (Trotti & Bliwise, 2010). Sometimes, symptoms are less specific, such as unrefreshing sleep, morning headache, or daytime sleepiness (see further below). There are several questionnaires used to screen for OSA in the general population. Many of these focus on traditional risk factors for OSA such as BMI and neck circumference (Chung et al., 2008; Netzer, Stoohs, Netzer, Clark, & Strohl, 1999). Since these risk factors for OSA may not necessarily apply in the PD population, these questionnaires should not be used in isolation to screen for OSA in PD until further studies to validate them are available. As for PSG, the gold standard is in-lab (observed) sleep testing. Home sleep studies (HSTs) can also be done and sometimes are mandated due to insurance company rules. Unattended portal sleep studies, usually in the form of HSTs, typically measure airflow, respiratory effort, and oximetry but do not include EEG leads and do not therefore capture arousals. HST lacks sensitivity for mild OSA in PD (Gros et al., 2015) and likely underestimates OSA in part because the arousals used to define obstructive respiratory events may not be captured. In PD patients with OSA, respiratory events may be more likely to be associated with arousals rather than desaturation (Diederich et al., 2005; Mery et al., 2017). HST may be particularly insensitive in PD patients with more severe motor manifestations (Gros et al., 2015). When HST is positive for OSA, it is accurate, but a negative HST in the setting of high suspicion for OSA in PD should prompt an in-lab study.

Epidemiology

Data indicate that individuals with PD are not at an increased risk of OSA as compared with the general population (Diederich, Rufra, Pieri, Hipp, & Vaillant, 2013; Trotti & Bliwise, 2010), and OSA is also not more severe in PD compared with the general population (Nieto et al., 2000; Redline, Min, Shahar, Rapoport, & O'Connor, 2005; Trotti & Bliwise, 2010). Rather, it is likely that the risk factors for OSA in PD are just different. Autonomic dysfunction in PD has been postulated to contribute to upper airway dysfunction and abnormal airway muscle coordination in PD (Zhang et al., 2016).

OSA, defined liberally as an AHI > 5/hour, may be present in up to 76% of individuals with PD (S. Chung et al., 2013). In another study using a cutoff of AHI $\geq$ 10, the prevalence was 55% (Neikrug et al., 2013). If more conservative criteria are used, in accordance with International Classification of Sleep Disorders (American Academy of Sleep Medicine, 2014), the prevalence of at least moderate OSA (AHI >15) was 22.4% (Nomura, Inoue, Kobayashi, Namba, & Nakashima, 2013), and severe OSA (AHI > 30) occurred in 17.9% in another study (Cochen De Cock et al., 2014). OSA may be more likely to occur in PD patients with more advanced disease (Cochen De Cock et al., 2010) but certainly can be seen in early

PD, in over one-third of PD patients (Joy et al., 2014; Prudon, Duncan, Khoo, Yarnall, & Anderson, 2014).

Some studies suggest that PD patients may be more likely to have central sleep apneas as compared with non-PD comparators (Valko, Hauser, Sommerauer, Werth, & Baumann, 2014), but this is not a consistent finding across studies (Cochen De Cock et al., 2010; Diederich et al., 2005; Yong, Fook-Chong, Pavanni, Lim, & Tan, 2011). It is possible that dopamine agonist use is associated with central apneas (Valko et al., 2014), although whether this is causative or confounding by indication is not clear.

REM sleep behavior disorder (RBD) may be a risk factor for OSA in PD, although data on this are conflicting. One study among 46 PD patients indicated that PD patients with polysomnographically-confirmed RBD may be particularly susceptible to OSA (Zhang et al., 2016). Among those with RBD, OSA, as defined by AHI > 5, occurred in 51.4% compared with 9.1% among those without RBD. Of note, those with RBD had similar REM-AHI compared with those without RBD. On the other hand, another study proposed that increased muscle tone during REM sleep, as is seen in RBD, could actually be protective against OSA in PD (Gong et al., 2014). One of the largest studies (Sixel-Doring, Trautmann, Mollenhauer, & Trenkwalder, 2011) of 457 with PD evaluated for RBD did not find an increased risk of sleep-disordered breathing (SDB) in PD patients with RBD versus those without, but AHI was not presented in that study. See Chapter 5 for more on RBD in PD patients and its implications.

Etiology and differential diagnosis

As mentioned, individuals with PD are not at an increased risk of OSA as compared with the general population. Rather, it is likely that the risk factors for OSA in PD are just different. For example, in addition to risk for upper airway obstruction, restrictive pulmonary function may be more likely in PD, perhaps due to thoracic muscle rigidity (Monteiro, Souza-Machado, Valderramas, & Melo, 2012; Sabate, Rodriguez, Mendez, Enriquez, & Gonzalez, 1996), changes in posture, and possibly even abnormal movements in the upper airway muscles analogous to tremor (4–8 Hz oscillations in upper airway muscles) (Schiffman, 1985; Vincken & Cosio, 1985). In one study the hypothesis was tested that serotonergic denervation predisposes PD patients to OSA, but the data did not support this (Lelieveld et al., 2012). In addition, individuals with PD have abnormal physiologic response to hypercapnia (Seccombe et al., 2011).

When arousals occur as a result of obstructive events in PD, they may be associated with vocalizations or movements that can mimic the dream enactment seen in REM sleep behavior disorder (RBD) (Iranzo & Santamaria, 2005). OSA is indeed on the differential of paroxysmal nocturnal behaviors in Parkinson's disease (Manni, Terzaghi, Repetto, Zangaglia, & Pacchetti, 2010).

Consequences and complications

The consequences of OSA in PD are likely at a minimum similar to those seen in the general population, namely increased risk of cardiovascular events, depression, and cognitive dysfunction (Diaz et al., 2014; Smith et al., 2002).

Excessive daytime sleepiness (EDS) is a common daytime consequence of OSA. EDS is common in PD (see also Chapter 12 on EDS in PD). It is multifactorial and could be a manifestation of underlying neurodegeneration. Therefore, it is not entirely surprising that many studies have not shown a relationship between SDB and EDS in PD (Cochen De Cock et al., 2014; Neikrug et al., 2013; Nomura et al., 2013; Prudon et al., 2014; Trotti & Bliwise, 2010), although a few have, and there are accumulating data that OSA may be a treatable etiology for EDS at least in some patients with PD. In one study, PD patients with an AHI $\geq$ 5 had greater EDS compared with those with AHI < 5 (Norlinah et al., 2009). An objective correlate of that is that PD patients with higher AHI had a shorter mean sleep latency (Chung et al., 2013; Cochen De Cock et al., 2014; Poryazova, Benninger, Waldvogel, & Bassetti, 2010; Yong et al., 2011). A study of 67 PD patients found 47 with OSA, with mean AHI of 27.1. There was a significant association between AHI and Epworth Sleepiness Scale (ESS) score after adjusting for age, sex, Hoehn and Yahr stage, and levodopa equivalent dose (Mery et al., 2017).

As for the consequences of SDB on cognition in PD, OSA has been independently associated with cognitive dysfunction in PD in several studies (Harmell et al., 2016; Mery et al., 2017; Neikrug et al., 2013). A study of 67 PD patients found 47 with OSA, with mean AHI of 27.1. Montreal Cognitive Assessment (MoCA) score was inversely related to OSA severity and remained significantly associated with AHI after adjusting for age and sex, as well as levodopa equivalents and ESS. Interestingly, MoCA was inversely associated with respiratory arousals but not intermittent hypoxia (Mery et al., 2017).

In the general population, OSA is associated with sympathetic overactivation, which may explain the increased prevalence of hypertension and cardiovascular events in individuals with OSA. The relationship between autonomic dysfunction and OSA in PD is complex. PD patients may not be more likely to have cardiovascular events as compared with the general population, but there are no strong data to indicate that PD patients are somehow protected from the adverse consequences of SDB (Nomura et al., 2013). PD patients with untreated OSA may have more autonomic symptoms than PD patients with treated OSA (Izzi et al., 2018). Autonomic dysfunction in PD also alters the response to obstructive events in PD: PD patients have a blunted response to apneas as compared with non-PD comparators, perhaps due to sympathetic dysfunction in PD (Valko, Hauser, Werth, Waldvogel, & Baumann, 2012).

Management

The main recommended treatment for OSA and other SDB in PD is positive airway pressure (PAP) (Patil, Ayappa, Caples, Kimoff, Patel, & Harrod, 2019a, 2019b).

Unfortunately, PAP is not well tolerated in many patients, and this certainly applies to patients with PD (Terzaghi et al., 2017). There are a few strategies that may improve PAP tolerance (Ballard, Gay, & Strollo, 2007; Patil et al., 2019a, 2019b). While these have not been specifically tested in PD patients, they are still of potential utility. Mask optimization is obviously critical, and several masks may have to be tried before a comfortable one is identified. Heat humidification to help with nasal dryness and nasal therapy to help with nasal congestion may also be useful. Other techniques include instructing the patient to wear the PAP during the day while awake, and educating the patient to practice relaxation techniques may be of benefit. A study in non-PD individuals indicates that adjustment of the type of positive airway pressure administered, namely use of flexible bilevel positive airway pressure instead of continuous positive airway pressure (CPAP) may improve compliance (Ballard et al., 2007). This deserves study in PD.

There are limited data on the effectiveness of CPAP on treatment of symptoms in PD patients with OSA. What data are available indicate that when CPAP is effectively used, it can improve sleep quality, sleepiness, and other symptoms. In one randomized trial of CPAP for OSA in PD, CPAP use was associated with reduced AHI and improved mean sleep latency (Neikrug et al., 2014).

Consistent use of CPAP is associated with improvements in cognition in the general population and in Alzheimer's' disease, but this has yet to be conclusively demonstrated in PD. One trial of 38 PD patients with OSA randomized to either placebo or therapeutic CPAP attempted to test this (Harmell et al., 2016). A benefit of CPAP on OSA could not be demonstrated on a comprehensive panel of neuropsychological testing, but the small sample size may have limited power to detect a difference. In an observational study of 67 PD patients, 48 were found to have OSA, and of those, 21 received CPAP therapy consistently and were compared with 21 with OSA who did not have an adequate trial of CPAP treatment. At 6-month follow-up, MoCA score had significantly improved in the PD patients with OSA treated with CPAP but not in the OSA patients not treated (Kaminska et al., 2018).

There are few data to guide treatment of OSA in PD patients who do not tolerate CPAP. Oral appliances are considered better than no therapy at all in the general population with OSA (Ramar et al., 2015).

Illustrative case in context

The patient in the case presented with daytime sleepiness. There was a history suggestive of OSA, and this was confirmed on PSG. He underwent CPAP titration. He had significant difficulty complying with consistent CPAP use, but after multiple attempts, and with trials of varies masks, he ultimately became accustomed to it and could wear it on average 5–6 hours/night. On follow-up 6 months later, he reported significant improvement in daytime sleepiness. His repeat ESS score was 8. His wife reported she was sleeping better too now that his snoring had been eliminated.

Many PD patients with OSA do not tolerate CPAP, but CPAP tolerance increases over time in some patients. While not all patients with PD and OSA have an improvement in their EDS after CPAP use, many patients do, and concerted efforts to achieve adequate CPAP therapy in PD are needed.

References

American Academy of Sleep Medicine. (2014). *International classification of sleep disorders* (3rd ed.). Darien, IL: American Academy of Sleep Medicine.

American Academy of Sleep Medicine. (April 2018). *The AASM manual for the scoring of sleep and associated events: Rules, terminology and technical specifications.*

Ballard, R. D., Gay, P. C., & Strollo, P. J. (2007). Interventions to improve compliance in sleep apnea patients previously non-compliant with continuous positive airway pressure. *Journal of Clinical Sleep Medicine: Official Publication of the American Academy of Sleep Medicine, 3*(7), 706−712.

Chung, S., Bohnen, N. I., Albin, R. L., Frey, K. A., Muller, M. L., & Chervin, R. D. (2013). Insomnia and sleepiness in Parkinson disease: Associations with symptoms and comorbidities. *Journal of Clinical Sleep Medicine: Official Publication of the American Academy of Sleep Medicine, 9*(11), 1131−1137.

Chung, F., Yegneswaran, B., Liao, P., Chung, S. A., Vairavanathan, S., Islam, S., et al. (2008). STOP questionnaire: A tool to screen patients for obstructive sleep apnea. *Anesthesiology, 108*(5), 812−821.

Cochen De Cock, V., Abouda, M., Leu, S., Oudiette, D., Roze, E., Vidailhet, M., et al. (2010). Is obstructive sleep apnea a problem in Parkinson's disease? *Sleep Medicine, 11*(3), 247−252.

Cochen De Cock, V., Bayard, S., Jaussent, I., Charif, M., Grini, M., Langenier, M. C., et al. (2014). Daytime sleepiness in Parkinson's disease: A reappraisal. *PLoS One, 9*(9), e107278.

Diaz, K., Faverio, P., Hospenthal, A., Restrepo, M. I., Amuan, M. E., & Pugh, M. J. (2014). Obstructive sleep apnea is associated with higher healthcare utilization in elderly patients. *Annals of Thoracic Medicine, 9*(2), 92−98.

Diederich, N. J., Rufra, O., Pieri, V., Hipp, G., & Vaillant, M. (2013). Lack of polysomno-graphic Non-REM sleep changes in early Parkinson's disease. *Movement Disorders: Official Journal of the Movement Disorder Society, 28*(10), 1443−1446.

Diederich, N. J., Vaillant, M., Leischen, M., Mancuso, G., Golinval, S., Nati, R., et al. (2005). Sleep apnea syndrome in Parkinson's disease. A case-control study in 49 patients. *Movement Disorders: Official Journal of the Movement Disorder Society, 20*(11), 1413−1418.

Gong, Y., Xiong, K. P., Mao, C. J., Shen, Y., Hu, W. D., Huang, J. Y., et al. (2014). Clinical manifestations of Parkinson disease and the onset of rapid eye movement sleep behavior disorder. *Sleep Medicine, 15*(6), 647−653.

Gros, P., Mery, V. P., Lafontaine, A. L., Robinson, A., Benedetti, A., Kimoff, R. J., et al. (2015). Diagnosis of obstructive sleep apnea in Parkinson's disease patients: Is unattended portable monitoring a suitable tool? *Parkinson's Disease, 2015*, 258418.

Harmell, A. L., Neikrug, A. B., Palmer, B. W., Avanzino, J. A., Liu, L., Maglione, J. E., et al. (2016). Obstructive sleep apnea and cognition in Parkinson's disease. *Sleep Medicine, 21*, 28−34.

Iranzo, A., & Santamaria, J. (2005). Severe obstructive sleep apnea/hypopnea mimicking REM sleep behavior disorder. *Sleep, 28*(2), 203−206.

Izzi, F., Placidi, F., Liguori, C., Lauretti, B., Marfia, G. A., Pisani, A., et al. (2018). Does continuous positive airway pressure treatment affect autonomic nervous system in patients with severe obstructive sleep apnea? *Sleep Medicine, 42*, 68−72.

Joy, S. P., Sinha, S., Pal, P. K., Panda, S., Philip, M., & Taly, A. B. (2014). Alterations in Polysomnographic (PSG) profile in drug-naive Parkinson's disease. *Annals of Indian Academy of Neurology, 17*(3), 287−291.

Kaminska, M., Mery, V. P., Lafontaine, A. L., Robinson, A., Benedetti, A., Gros, P., et al. (2018). Change in cognition and other non-motor symptoms with obstructive sleep apnea treatment in Parkinson disease. *Journal of Clinical Sleep Medicine: Official Publication of the American Academy of Sleep Medicine, 14*(5), 819−828.

Lelieveld, I. M., Muller, M. L., Bohnen, N. I., Koeppe, R. A., Chervin, R. D., Frey, K. A., et al. (2012). The role of serotonin in sleep disordered breathing associated with Parkinson disease: A correlative [11C]DASB PET imaging study. *PLoS One, 7*(7), e40166.

Manni, R., Terzaghi, M., Repetto, A., Zangaglia, R., & Pacchetti, C. (2010). Complex paroxysmal nocturnal behaviors in Parkinson's disease. *Movement Disorders: Official Journal of the Movement Disorder Society, 25*(8), 985−990.

Mery, V. P., Gros, P., Lafontaine, A. L., Robinson, A., Benedetti, A., Kimoff, R. J., et al. (2017). Reduced cognitive function in patients with Parkinson disease and obstructive sleep apnea. *Neurology, 88*(12), 1120−1128.

Monteiro, L., Souza-Machado, A., Valderramas, S., & Melo, A. (2012). The effect of levodopa on pulmonary function in Parkinson's disease: A systematic review and meta-analysis. *Clinical Therapeutics, 34*(5), 1049−1055.

Neikrug, A. B., Liu, L., Avanzino, J. A., Maglione, J. E., Natarajan, L., Bradley, L., et al. (2014). Continuous positive airway pressure improves sleep and daytime sleepiness in patients with Parkinson disease and sleep apnea. *Sleep, 37*(1), 177−185.

Neikrug, A. B., Maglione, J. E., Liu, L., Natarajan, L., Avanzino, J. A., Corey-Bloom, J., et al. (2013). Effects of sleep disorders on the non-motor symptoms of Parkinson disease. *Journal of Clinical Sleep Medicine: Official Publication of the American Academy of Sleep Medicine, 9*(11), 1119−1129.

Netzer, N. C., Stoohs, R. A., Netzer, C. M., Clark, K., & Strohl, K. P. (1999). Using the Berlin Questionnaire to identify patients at risk for the sleep apnea syndrome. *Annals of Internal Medicine, 131*(7), 485−491.

Nieto, F. J., Young, T. B., Lind, B. K., Shahar, E., Samet, J. M., Redline, S., et al. (2000). Association of sleep-disordered breathing, sleep apnea, and hypertension in a large community-based study. Sleep Heart Health Study. *The Journal of the American Medical Association, 283*(14), 1829−1836.

Nomura, T., Inoue, Y., Kobayashi, M., Namba, K., & Nakashima, K. (2013). Characteristics of obstructive sleep apnea in patients with Parkinson's disease. *Journal of the Neurological Sciences, 327*(1−2), 22−24.

Norlinah, M. I., Afidah, K. N., Noradina, A. T., Shamsul, A. S., Hamidon, B. B., Sahathevan, R., et al. (2009). Sleep disturbances in Malaysian patients with Parkinson's disease using polysomnography and PDSS. *Parkinsonism & Related Disorders, 15*(9), 670−674.

Patil, S. P., Ayappa, I. A., Caples, S. M., Kimoff, R. J., Patel, S. R., & Harrod, C. G. (2019a). Treatment of adult obstructive sleep apnea with positive airway pressure: An American Academy of Sleep medicine Clinical Practice Guideline. *Journal of Clinical Sleep Medicine: Official Publication of the American Academy of Sleep Medicine.*

Patil, S. P., Ayappa, I. A., Caples, S. M., Kimoff, R. J., Patel, S. R., & Harrod, C. G. (2019b). Treatment of adult obstructive sleep apnea with positive airway pressure: An American Academy of Sleep Medicine systematic review, meta-analysis, and GRADE assessment. *Journal of Clinical Sleep Medicine: Official Publication of the American Academy of Sleep Medicine, 15*(2), 335−343.

Poryazova, R., Benninger, D., Waldvogel, D., & Bassetti, C. L. (2010). Excessive daytime sleepiness in Parkinson's disease: Characteristics and determinants. *European Neurology, 63*(3), 129−135.

Prudon, B., Duncan, G. W., Khoo, T. K., Yarnall, A. J., & Anderson, K. N. (2014). Primary sleep disorder prevalence in patients with newly diagnosed Parkinson's disease. *Movement Disorders: Official Journal of the Movement Disorder Society, 29*(2), 259−262.

Ramar, K., Dort, L. C., Katz, S. G., Lettieri, C. J., Harrod, C. G., Thomas, S. M., et al. (2015). Clinical practice guideline for the treatment of obstructive sleep apnea and snoring with oral appliance therapy: An update for 2015. *Journal of Clinical Sleep Medicine: Official Publication of the American Academy of Sleep Medicine, 11*(7), 773−827.

Redline, S., Min, N. I., Shahar, E., Rapoport, D., & O'Connor, G. (2005). Polysomnographic predictors of blood pressure and hypertension: Is one index best? *Sleep, 28*(9), 1122−1130.

Sabate, M., Rodriguez, M., Mendez, E., Enriquez, E., & Gonzalez, I. (1996). Obstructive and restrictive pulmonary dysfunction increases disability in Parkinson disease. *Archives of Physical Medicine and Rehabilitation, 77*(1), 29−34.

Schiffman, P. L. (1985). A "saw-tooth" pattern in Parkinson's disease. *Chest, 87*(1), 124−126.

Seccombe, L. M., Giddings, H. L., Rogers, P. G., Corbett, A. J., Hayes, M. W., Peters, M. J., et al. (2011). Abnormal ventilatory control in Parkinson's disease–further evidence for non-motor dysfunction. *Respiratory Physiology & Neurobiology, 179*(2−3), 300−304.

Sixel-Doring, F., Trautmann, E., Mollenhauer, B., & Trenkwalder, C. (2011). Associated factors for REM sleep behavior disorder in Parkinson disease. *Neurology, 77*(11), 1048−1054.

Smith, R., Ronald, J., Delaive, K., Walld, R., Manfreda, J., & Kryger, M. H. (2002). What are obstructive sleep apnea patients being treated for prior to this diagnosis? *Chest, 121*(1), 164−172.

Terzaghi, M., Spelta, L., Minafra, B., Rustioni, V., Zangaglia, R., Pacchetti, C., et al. (2017). Treating sleep apnea in Parkinson's disease with C-PAP: Feasibility concerns and effects on cognition and alertness. *Sleep Medicine, 33*, 114−118.

Trotti, L. M., & Bliwise, D. L. (2010). No increased risk of obstructive sleep apnea in Parkinson's disease. *Movement Disorders: Official Journal of the Movement Disorder Society, 25*(13), 2246−2249.

Valko, P. O., Hauser, S., Sommerauer, M., Werth, E., & Baumann, C. R. (2014). Observations on sleep-disordered breathing in idiopathic Parkinson's disease. *PLoS One, 9*(6), e100828.

Valko, P. O., Hauser, S., Werth, E., Waldvogel, D., & Baumann, C. R. (2012). Heart rate variability in patients with idiopathic Parkinson's disease with and without obstructive sleep apnea syndrome. *Parkinsonism & Related Disorders, 18*(5), 525−531.

Vincken, W., & Cosio, M. G. (1985). "Saw-tooth" pattern in the flow-volume loop. *Chest, 88*(3), 480−481.

Yong, M. H., Fook-Chong, S., Pavanni, R., Lim, L. L., & Tan, E. K. (2011). Case control polysomnographic studies of sleep disorders in Parkinson's disease. *PLoS One, 6*(7), e22511.

Zhang, L. Y., Liu, W. Y., Kang, W. Y., Yang, Q., Wang, X. Y., Ding, J. Q., et al. (2016). Association of rapid eye movement sleep behavior disorder with sleep-disordered breathing in Parkinson's disease. *Sleep Medicine, 20*, 110−115.

Circadian rhythm abnormalities

Illustrative case

A 67-year-old man has had Parkinson's disease (PD) for 3 years. His main motor symptom is tremor, with mild stiffness, and his motor symptoms are well controlled on levodopa. He takes levodopa 150 mg three times a day, with the time of the first dose varying dramatically from 8:00 a.m. to 12:00 p.m., depending on what time he wakes up. Related to the latter, he complains of trouble falling asleep. On detailed sleep history, he reveals that while most of his household members go to bed at 10 p.m., he does not feel ready to sleep at that time. Sometimes he will try to, and he simply cannot. Instead, he either lies awake in bed, or gets up and watches TV, and does not get sleepy until 2 a.m. Once he falls asleep, he sleeps well, and feels like he could sleep until 10 or 11 a.m., though his wife often wakes him up at 8 a.m. so that they can have breakfast together. On days that she does this, he feels very sleepy at around 1:00 or 2:00 p.m. and naps in the afternoon. His history further reveals he has followed this sleep pattern (of sleeping 2 a.m. and ideally until 10 or 11 a.m.) ever since he began working at a casino at age 22, and this pattern persists now, even though he retired 3 years earlier.

Overview
Definition

Broadly speaking, circadian rhythms are the endogenous cycles that have a periodicity of about 24 hours. These cycles are biological/physiological, but with behavioral manifestations as well. The latter, the behavioral manifestations of circadian rhythms, is called the "chronotype." The sleep—wake cycle is one of the best characterized circadian rhythms in living organism. Other examples include circadian changes in the hypothalamic—pituitary access, and autonomic function (blood pressure and heart rate). Circadian rhythms are synchronized with the light—dark cycle. Circadian oscillations of the sleep—wake cycle are genetically determined in humans. In humans, the circadian cycle is 24.18 hours in duration, and this is normally relatively stable across the lifespan (Czeisler et al., 1999).

Disorders of Sleep and Wakefulness in Parkinson's Disease. https://doi.org/10.1016/B978-0-323-67374-7.00009-2

Circadian rhythm sleep—wake disorders result from "misalignment of endogenous circadian rhythm and the external environment" (American Academy of Sleep Medicine, 2014). According to the American Academy of Sleep Medicine International Classification of Sleep Disorders—version 3, the general criteria for a circadian rhythm sleep—wake cycle disorder include "a chronic or recurrent pattern of sleep disruption primarily due to alteration of the endogenous circadian timing system and the sleep—wake schedule desired or required," and leading to clinically significant distress as well as either trouble initiating or maintaining sleep (insomnia) and/or daytime sleepiness. Circadian rhythm disorders that may be seen in PD include delayed sleep phase, in which the phase of major sleep is shifted forward, such that the natural sleep time and wakeup time occur later than societal norms/what is often desired. In contrast, with advanced sleep phase, the sleep/wakeup time is advanced, occurring earlier.

In PD, in addition to the occurrence of circadian rhythm disorders, several abnormalities of circadian rhythm have been identified. To understand these, a basic overview of definitions and measures of circadian rhythm is shown in Table 9.1 (Bjorvatn & Pallesen, 2009; Fifel, 2017; Videnovic, Lazar, Barker, & Overeem, 2014). Changes in core body temperature are a core measure of circadian rhythm. Core body temperature typically peaks in the late afternoon/early evening, and reaches the nadir (lowest point) in the early morning. Sleep onset typically occurs as body temperature begins to decline, and arousal from sleep typically occurs about 2 hours after the nadir is reached. Similarly increases in the secretion of melatonin, a hormone intricately related to circadian function, starts to increase at the onset of darkness, peaks around midnight, and gradually falls subsequently. Thus, in a pattern similar to the relationship between sleep and core body temperature, sleep occurs as melatonin levels peak and ends as melatonin levels reach their nadir.

Zeitgebers are environmental cues that can influence, and indeed regulate, circadian rhythm (Bjorvatn & Pallesen, 2009). Natural environmental light is the most potent zeitgeber.

Epidemiology

There are no robust data on the epidemiology of circadian rhythm disorders in PD. However, several studies have identified abnormalities of circadian rhythm in PD. These studies are limited by small sample sizes.

Compared to non-PD controls, PD patients have a lower amplitude of hormone peaks related to circadian function, as well as alterations in expression of circadian genes (Breen et al., 2014; Cai, Liu, Sothern, Xu, & Chan, 2010; Videnovic, Noble et al., 2014). Although early studies indicated a possible phase advancement in circadian function in PD (Bordet et al., 2003; Fertl, Auff, Doppelbauer, & Waldhauser, 1991), there were methodological limitations to the study design that could have confounded those results, and several subsequent studies have not found that a phase advancement in circadian function in PD is present (Bolitho et al., 2014; Videnovic, Noble et al., 2014).

Table 9.1 Definitions, measures, and patterns relevant to circadian rhythm.

Measure	Comment
Core body temperature	Sleep onset typically occurs as body temperature begins to decline, and arousal from sleep typically occurs about 2 hours after the nadir is reached. In patients with stable circadian rhythm, core body temperature nadir can be estimated from history obtained from the patient.
Melatonin secretion	Increases at onset of darkness, peaks around midnight, and then starts to fall. Melatonin can be measured in plasma, saliva, or urine. Dim light melatonin onset is a commonly used measure; it is the time at which melatonin level reaches 2 pg/mL in plasma or 4 pg/mL in saliva. In another approach, serial sampling can occur and various parameters examined.
Zeitgebers ("time givers")	Environmental cues that can influence, and indeed regulate, circadian rhythm
Phase angle of entrainment	Relationship between the timing of the biological clock and the timing of an external time cue. This can be assessed for core body temperature, melatonin, gene expression, and other measures that reflect circadian rhythm
"Molecular clock": Gene expression	Gene expression and gene expression inhibition constitutes a core of the mammalian circadian clock. A complex but well-characterized set of genes function in an interconnected network of negative and positive transcription-related loops. Transcriptomic methods can be applied to measure the degree and patterns of gene expression at given times within the circadian cycle
Rest-activity rhythm (RAR) measurements	Rest and activity levels, as measured by actigraphy, offer a measure of circadian function that can be acquired over several days in the subject's natural environment. Rest-activity rhythm measures commonly used include the acrophase, or time of peak activity level, the amplitude of maximal activity, and the mesor (mean of activity fitted curve). Several other variables can be derived from several-day actigraphy

In a study of 20 PD patients compared to 15 non-PD age-matched controls, blood samples were acquired every 30 minutes over a 24 hour period and melatonin was measured (Videnovic, Noble et al., 2014). A lower maximal amplitude of melatonin secretion, and lower 24-hour area under the curve for circulating melatonin levels were found in the PD group compared to the non-PD group. Similar findings were seen in a study of 30 PD patients and compared to 15 non-PD controls in which blood was also sampled over a 24 hour period. Melatonin levels exhibited a significant time-dependent variation in the non-PD group, but not in the PD group (Breen et al., 2014). PD patients had a reduced area under the curve for melatonin, indicating reduced circulating melatonin levels, but also a reduced melatonin nadir. In addition, PD patients had increased area under the curve for cortisol, increased amplitude, and increased acrophase. As for "clock genes," there was a lack of time-dependent variation in the PD group, compared to non-PD controls, for expression of the gene *Bmal1*. Similar findings were seen in a study of expression of clock genes in the peripheral leukocytes of 17 PD patients compared to non-PD controls (Cai et al., 2010). In this study, *Bmal1* expression was also found to be reduced in the PD group. Abnormal epigenetics (methylation patterns of promoters of clock genes) in PD has been demonstrated that may offer a potential mechanism for this (Lin et al., 2012). Reduced dopamine levels in PD may mediate abnormal expression patterns of *Bmal1*, as dopamine is known to regulate *Bmal1* expression.

In a study of 29 PD patients and 28 age-matched non-PD controls that investigated melatonin secretion (Bolitho et al., 2014), and different from some of the previously mentioned studies (Breen et al., 2014; Cai et al., 2010; Videnovic, Noble et al., 2014), environmental light exposure (which could alter melatonin dynamics) was fixed at 30 lux. Saliva samples were collected every 30 minutes for 6 hours before habitual sleep onset time and until 2 hours after. Salivary melatonin was measured. Dim light melatonin onset did not differ in the PD compared to the non-PD group. The medicated PD group had a longer phase angle compared to the non-PD group, but this difference was not found in comparing the unmedicated PD group to the non-PD group. As for the area under the curve for melatonin, the medicated PD patients had twice the level as compared to unmedicated patients, and also compared to controls. Here again, the unmedicated group did not differ significantly from the non-PD group. The medicated PD group had longer sleep latencies in relation to their dim light melatonin onset. The prolonged phase angle of entrainment of the melatonin rhythm was interpreted as indicating that there may be "uncoupling" of circadian and sleep–wake regulation in PD (Bolitho et al., 2014). The possibility of "melatonin resistance" in PD was also proposed, and this requires further study. Finally, these results indicate that exogenous dopaminergic therapy increases melatonin secretion, which is important to keep in mind in interpretation of any study of circadian function in PD.

Rest-activity rhythm (RAR) using wrist actigraphy have also been used to study circadian function in PD. Studies of RAR using actigraphy in PD patients have shown decreased diurnal activity and increased nocturnal activity (Van Hilten et al., 1994, 1993; Whitehead, Davies, Playfer, & Turnbull, 2008). For example, in one study of RAR, wrist actigraphy was applied in 50 PD patients and 29 healthy controls (Whitehead et al., 2008). Compared to controls, PD patients had lower peak activity levels and lower amplitude of activity, likely reflecting the impaired mobility (with relative paucity of movement) seen in PD. PD patients also showed greater variability from one 24 hour period to the next, indicating less predictability from 1 day to the next.

In some PD patients, diurnal patterns to motor function are seen as well, with worsening motor function and reduced levodopa responsiveness as the day progresses, despite stable drug doses (Bonuccelli et al., 2000; Nyholm, Lennernas, Johansson, Estrada, & Aquilonius, 2010; Videnovic, Noble et al., 2014). Abnormalities in circadian rhythm may account for some of these findings. Likely also accounting for some of the diurnal variations seen in PD is that levodopa absorption takes longer at night and when taken in supine position (Nyholm et al., 2010). In addition, autonomic dysfunction in PD manifests with abnormalities in the circadian rhythmicity of parameters such as diurnal blood pressure, postprandial hypotension, and heart rate variability (Kallio et al., 2000; Kallio et al., 2004; Senard, Chamontin, Rascol, & Montastruc, 1992).

Etiology and differential diagnosis

The suprachiasmatic nucleus is the structure from which the endogenous circadian rhythm originates and is driven (Videnovic, Noble et al., 2014). It is located in the hypothalamus. Lesions to this nucleus can eliminate circadian rhythm all together (Bjorvatn & Pallesen, 2009). Function of the suprachiasmatic nucleus is affected by various inputs, including projections from the retina. The monosynaptic retino-hypothalamic tract relays light input via photoreceptors, retinal cells that contain the light-sensing pigment, melanopsin. In addition, there are inhibitory projections, mediated by melatonin, from the pineal gland to the suprachiasmatic nucleus. In turn, GABAergic projections from the suprachiasmatic nucleus inhibit melatonin production by the pineal gland (Kalsbeek, Cutrera, Van Heerikhuize, Van Der Vliet, & Buijs, 1999). There is thus a feedback loop in place such that, under normal conditions, light leads to suprachiasmatic nucleus activation and melatonin inhibition during wakefulness, and in the dark, the suprachiasmatic nucleus activity is suppressed, during periods of melatonin production. Small studies have found that Lewy body pathology (the pathologic hallmark of PD) affects the suprachiasmatic nucleus in PD (De Pablo-Fernandez, Courtney, Warner, & Holton, 2018), and hypothalamic atrophy is seen in PD as well (Breen et al., 2016). In a study of 12 PD patients and 12 non-PD controls, hypothalamic volume was measured on MRI and found to be significantly reduced in PD compared to controls. Importantly, serum melatonin levels (measured in blood samples obtained every 90 minutes over a 24 hour period) were significantly associated with hypothalamic gray matter volume. Hypothalamic neuronal dysfunction (and/or loss) in PD may in turn account for some of the circadian abnormalities seen in PD (Breen et al., 2014; Videnovic, Lazar et al., 2014; Videnovic, Noble et al., 2014). Retinal abnormalities in PD may further contribute to circadian abnormalities (Fifel, 2017). Postmortem examination of retina from six donors with history of PD, and compared to five non-PD controls, revealed a reduction in melanopsin-containing retinal ganglion cells in the PD group (Ortuno-Lizaran et al., 2018). A reduction in the complexity of the plexus of cells, as well as changes in the morphology of cells seen in the retinas of the PD patients compared to control was reported. The small sample size limits conclusions that can be drawn, but provides intriguing possibilities to explore regarding contributors to the pathophysiology of circadian dysfunction in PD.

Dopamine plays a central role in circadian function (Fifel, 2017; Mendoza & Challet, 2014). Dopamine is subject to the effects of circadian rhythm, and in turn exerts effects on the circadian system. Dopamine modulates physiological responses resulting from retinal activation by light. Indeed, dopamine deficiency has been hypothesized to contribute to the circadian dysfunction seen in PD (Breen et al., 2014; Fifel, 2017).The effect of PD medications in increasing melatonin secretion (Bolitho et al., 2014) is critical to account for in interpretation of any studies on circadian function in medicated PD patients. In addition, exogenous dopamine may exert effects on expression of clock genes in the suprachiasmatic nucleus, and this may also be a critical factorcontributing to circadian disruption in PD (Fifel, 2017).

Consequences and complications

Circadian variations in dopamine release, as well as circadian changes in exogenous levodopa exposure and effect, may account for some of the diurnal variations in symptoms that PD patients experience. A small study of three PD patients and three non-PD controls measured dopamine and its metabolites in CSF (Poceta, Parsons, Engelland, & Kripke, 2009). The results indicated that dopamine release is maximal in the mornings around 10 a.m.; what contribution this has to "sleep benefit," the relatively better motor function some PD patients find after sleep and especially in the mornings, is not clear. See Chapter 11 for more on sleep benefit.

Circadian abnormalities may be seen in relation to manifestations of other non-motor signs and symptoms in PD. Indeed, circadian dysfunction is seen in PD patients with excessive daytime sleepiness (EDS), a common and disabling manifestation of PD. In a study of 20 PD patients, the 12 with EDS had significantly lower amplitude of melatonin rhythm and 24-hour area under the curve compared to the 8 without (Videnovic, Noble et al., 2014). Whether abnormalities in melatonin secretion or other circadian functions directly cause daytime sleepiness, or whether neurodegeneration of specific neuroanatomic regions, combined with physiologic abnormalities, contributes to both circadian dysfunction and daytime sleepiness, is not clear but deserves further study. See Chapter 12 for more on EDS in PD.

Abnormalities in rest activity levels (RAR) may be a manifestation of other non-motor symptoms in PD as well. For example, as discussed in Chapter 4, PD patients with hallucinations have greater nocturnal activity levels, reflecting disturbed sleep (Whitehead et al., 2008).

Urine production also follows a circadian rhythm, such that 25% or less of 24 hour urine output is normally produced at night (Batla, Phe, De Min, & Panicker, 2016). This may result from effects of melatonin and vasopressin, as well as circadian differences in sodium and free water handling in the renal tubules. There are few data on circadian rhythmicity of urine production in PD, but abnormalities in this rhythm could, in theory, account for the polyuria seen in many PD patients who in turn report disrupted sleep. Whether melatonin supplementation could benefit nocturia in PD deserves further study, based on results of a small study of 20 older men with benign prostatic hypertrophy (without PD) (Drake, Mills, & Noble, 2004).

Management

Treatment of circadian disorders in PD is similar to treatment of these disorders in the general population (Bjorvatn & Pallesen, 2009). Treatment is best achieved by a trained sleep specialist, where available. Having the patient complete a 2-week sleep diary helps to provide information on natural bedtime and wakeup time, which in turn guides therapy. Bright light exposure before the nadir of core body temperature shifts the phase forward, whereas bright light exposure after the nadir advances the phase forward. This can be used to manipulate circadian rhythm. For example, in a patient with delayed sleep phase, bright light exposure, to either sunlight or portable lamps (at 10,000 lux), for 30—45 minutes, strategically timed based on the patient's history of typical wakeup time, can be used to advance the sleep phase. This can be particularly effective when coupled with exogenous melatonin treatment administered in the early evening (5—7 hours before regular sleep onset time). On the other hand, in patients with advanced sleep phase, bright light exposure in the evening will help to shift the bedtime forward. Determining the timing of administration of bright light and/or melatonin is critical, as incorrect timing of these therapies can lead to exacerbation of circadian disorders.

In PD, what is often seen is an irregular sleep—wake rhythm, often exacerbated by EDS with irregular but prolonged daytime naps. In such cases, daytime stimulation with physical and social activities is necessary. Scheduled bedtime and wakeup times are necessary, and in select cases morning bright light exposure can be helpful. The role of bright light therapy in PD outside of a diagnosis of a circadian disorder is not clear. Preliminary data indicate that, as discussed in Chapter 1, bright light therapy can be effective for insomnia and EDS even in the absence of a diagnosable circadian disorder.

Illustrative case in context

In the case described, on initial impression it may seem as though this patient has sleep initiation insomnia. However, careful examination of his history indicates that instead, he has delayed sleep phase syndrome. In this syndrome, circadian rhythm is shifted forward such that the body "clock" is not following typical societal norms (or, in this case, household norms) for bedtime but rather is delayed several hours. This is not uncommon in shift workers and/or individuals who work jobs that require them to stay up late (and, as in this case, persists after the evening job ends). There are not data to indicate that delayed sleep phase is more common in PD than the general population, and its treatment in this case would follow typical protocols including early bright light exposure, timed to occur at, for example, 9 a.m. and gradually moved back (though kept within 2 hours of the estimated nadir of core body temperature). In addition, melatonin to be taken at, for example, 6:00 p.m. or 7:00 p.m. In patients with delayed sleep phase, as the shift in sleep is achieved with therapy, adjustment of PD medication timing may be required as well. In this case, his morning dose of levodopa would be timed earlier, if/when he starts to sleep earlier and wake up earlier.

References

American Academy of Sleep Medicine. (2014). *International classification of sleep disorders* (3rd ed.). Darien, IL: American Academy of Sleep Medicine.

Batla, A., Phe, V., De Min, L., & Panicker, J. N. (2016). Nocturia in Parkinson's disease: Why does it occur and how to manage? *Movement Disorders Clinical Practice, 3*(5), 443–451.

Bjorvatn, B., & Pallesen, S. (2009). A practical approach to circadian rhythm sleep disorders. *Sleep Medicine Reviews, 13*(1), 47–60.

Bolitho, S. J., Naismith, S. L., Rajaratnam, S. M., Grunstein, R. R., Hodges, J. R., Terpening, Z., et al. (2014). Disturbances in melatonin secretion and circadian sleep-wake regulation in Parkinson disease. *Sleep Medicine, 15*(3), 342–347.

Bonuccelli, U., Del Dotto, P., Lucetti, C., Petrozzi, L., Bernardini, S., Gambaccini, G., et al. (2000). Diurnal motor variations to repeated doses of levodopa in Parkinson's disease. *Clinical Neuropharmacology, 23*(1), 28–33.

Bordet, R., Devos, D., Brique, S., Touitou, Y., Guieu, J. D., Libersa, C., et al. (2003). Study of circadian melatonin secretion pattern at different stages of Parkinson's disease. *Clinical Neuropharmacology, 26*(2), 65–72.

Breen, D. P., Nombela, C., Vuono, R., Jones, P. S., Fisher, K., Burn, D. J., et al. (2016). Hypothalamic volume loss is associated with reduced melatonin output in Parkinson's disease. *Movement Disorders: Official Journal of the Movement Disorder Society, 31*(7), 1062–1066.

Breen, D. P., Vuono, R., Nawarathna, U., Fisher, K., Shneerson, J. M., Reddy, A. B., et al. (2014). Sleep and circadian rhythm regulation in early Parkinson disease. *JAMA Neurology, 71*(5), 589–595.

Cai, Y., Liu, S., Sothern, R. B., Xu, S., & Chan, P. (2010). Expression of clock genes Per1 and Bmal1 in total leukocytes in health and Parkinson's disease. *European Journal of Neurology, 17*(4), 550–554.

Czeisler, C. A., Duffy, J. F., Shanahan, T. L., Brown, E. N., Mitchell, J. F., Rimmer, D. W., et al. (1999). Stability, precision, and near-24-hour period of the human circadian pacemaker. *Science (New York, N.Y.), 284*(5423), 2177–2181.

De Pablo-Fernandez, E., Courtney, R., Warner, T. T., & Holton, J. L. (2018). A histologic study of the circadian system in Parkinson disease, multiple system Atrophy, and progressive supranuclear palsy. *JAMA Neurology, 75*(8), 1008–1012.

Drake, M. J., Mills, I. W., & Noble, J. G. (2004). Melatonin pharmacotherapy for nocturia in men with benign prostatic enlargement. *The Journal of Urology, 171*(3), 1199–1202.

Fertl, E., Auff, E., Doppelbauer, A., & Waldhauser, F. (1991). Circadian secretion pattern of melatonin in Parkinson's disease. *Journal of Neural Transmission - Parkinson's Disease & Dementia Section, 3*(1), 41–47.

Fifel, K. (2017). Alterations of the circadian system in Parkinson's disease patients. *Movement Disorders: Official Journal of the Movement Disorder Society, 32*(5), 682−692.

Kallio, M., Haapaniemi, T., Turkka, J., Suominen, K., Tolonen, U., Sotaniemi, K., et al. (2000). Heart rate variability in patients with untreated Parkinson's disease. *European Journal of Neurology, 7*(6), 667−672.

Kallio, M., Suominen, K., Haapaniemi, T., Sotaniemi, K., Myllyla, V. V., Astafiev, S., et al. (2004). Nocturnal cardiac autonomic regulation in Parkinson's disease. *Clinical Autonomic Research: Official Journal of the Clinical Autonomic Research Society, 14*(2), 119−124.

Kalsbeek, A., Cutrera, R. A., Van Heerikhuize, J. J., Van Der Vliet, J., & Buijs, R. M. (1999). GABA release from suprachiasmatic nucleus terminals is necessary for the light-induced inhibition of nocturnal melatonin release in the rat. *Neuroscience, 91*(2), 453−461.

Lin, Q., Ding, H., Zheng, Z., Gu, Z., Ma, J., Chen, L., et al. (2012). Promoter methylation analysis of seven clock genes in Parkinson's disease. *Neuroscience Letters, 507*(2), 147−150.

Mendoza, J., & Challet, E. (2014). Circadian insights into dopamine mechanisms. *Neuroscience, 282*, 230−242.

Nyholm, D., Lennernas, H., Johansson, A., Estrada, M., & Aquilonius, S. M. (2010). Circadian rhythmicity in levodopa pharmacokinetics in patients with Parkinson disease. *Clinical Neuropharmacology, 33*(4), 181−185.

Ortuno-Lizaran, I., Esquiva, G., Beach, T. G., Serrano, G. E., Adler, C. H., Lax, P., et al. (2018). Degeneration of human photosensitive retinal ganglion cells may explain sleep and circadian rhythms disorders in Parkinson's disease. *Acta Neuropathologica Communications, 6*(1), 90, 9018-0596-z.

Poceta, J. S., Parsons, L., Engelland, S., & Kripke, D. F. (2009). Circadian rhythm of CSF monoamines and hypocretin-1 in restless legs syndrome and Parkinson's disease. *Sleep Medicine, 10*(1), 129−133.

Senard, J. M., Chamontin, B., Rascol, A., & Montastruc, J. L. (1992). Ambulatory blood pressure in patients with Parkinson's disease without and with orthostatic hypotension. *Clinical Autonomic Research: Official Journal of the Clinical Autonomic Research Society, 2*(2), 99−104.

Van Hilten, B., Hoff, J. I., Middelkoop, H. A., van der Velde, E. A., Kerkhof, G. A., Wauquier, A., et al. (1994). Sleep disruption in Parkinson's disease. Assessment by continuous activity monitoring. *Archives of Neurology, 51*(9), 922−928.

Van Hilten, J. J., Hoogland, G., van der Velde, E. A., van Dijk, J. G., Kerkhof, G. A., & Roos, R. A. (1993). Quantitative assessment of parkinsonian patients by continuous wrist activity monitoring. *Clinical Neuropharmacology, 16*(1), 36−45.

Videnovic, A., Lazar, A. S., Barker, R. A., & Overeem, S. (2014). The clocks that time us'− circadian rhythms in neurodegenerative disorders. *Nature Reviews Neurology, 10*(12), 683−693.

Videnovic, A., Noble, C., Reid, K. J., Peng, J., Turek, F. W., Marconi, A., et al. (2014). Circadian melatonin rhythm and excessive daytime sleepiness in Parkinson disease. *JAMA Neurology, 71*(4), 463−469.

Whitehead, D. L., Davies, A. D., Playfer, J. R., & Turnbull, C. J. (2008). Circadian rest-activity rhythm is altered in Parkinson's disease patients with hallucinations. *Movement Disorders: Official Journal of the Movement Disorder Society, 23*(8), 1137−1145.

Nocturia

Illustrative case

A 72-year-old man with Parkinson's disease (PD) of 7 years duration reports that 2−3 years ago, he began having to get up at night to urinate, and in subsequent years this gradually increased such that he now gets up to urinate five times a night. This is very disruptive to his sleep and he reports feeling tired and cranky all day. He reports that he get into bed around 10 p.m. and is usually so exhausted that he falls straight to sleep. However, he wakes up at 1−2 a.m. with the urge to urinate, and then goes back to bed and falls asleep only to wake up 1−2 hours later again with the urge to urinate. He reports that during nighttime urination, he estimates similar amounts of urine output for each episode as he does for an episode of urination during the day. In regards to daytime urinary symptoms, he also has urinary frequency and sometimes has a sudden urge to urinate that occasionally (on three separate occasions in the past year) was associated with incontinence because there was not a bathroom nearby.

Overview
Definition

Nocturia is defined as the awakening at night to void, with the episode of micturition preceded and followed by sleep. The first consensus definition on nocturia required only a single episode a night for the designation of nocturia (Hashim et al., 2019). However, it was soon recognized that this was a problematic definition because not all episodes of nocturnal micturition are necessarily pathologic, and one or even two episodes of micturition a night may not be clinically significant and/or may not be considered, by patients, to be particularly bothersome or disruptive to their sleep. Thus, for practical purposes, nocturia in PD, as it relates to sleep disruption, can be defined as at least one episode of micturition preceded and followed by sleep that is bothersome to the patient.

The diagnosis of sleep-disruptive nocturia is made based on history. Bladder diaries, in which patients document the timing of micturition episodes in relation to sleep, may be helpful.

Disorders of Sleep and Wakefulness in Parkinson's Disease. https://doi.org/10.1016/B978-0-323-67374-7.00010-9

Nocturia may be comorbid with the related disorder of nocturnal polyuria. Polyuria is defined as the "passing of large volumes of urine during the main sleep phase" (Hashim et al., 2019). Nocturnal polyuria is designated when the volume of urine output at night is excessive. Nocturnal polyuria is defined when nocturnal urine output accounts for >20% of urine volume occurring over a 24 hour period.

Epidemiology

What data are available indicate that nocturia is more common in PD than in the general population. One study assessed nocturia via a questionnaire in 61 PD patients compared to 74 non-PD controls (Campos-Sousa et al., 2003). Nocturia was present in 63% of the PD patients compared to 32.8% of controls.

The prevalence of nocturia in PD varies according to the ascertainment method, with prevalence of 34%−86% reported (Barone et al., 2009; Batla, Phe, De Min, & Panicker, 2016; Sakakibara et al., 2001; Sammour et al., 2009; Winge, Skau, Stimpel, Nielsen, & Werdelin, 2006). Studies that have administered questionnaires specific to urinary symptoms have found higher prevalences (Sammour et al., 2009; Winge et al., 2006) than a study that screened for nocturia using semistructured interview in 1072 PD patients (Barone et al., 2009). Nocturia is more common in older patients (Campos-Sousa et al., 2003). Some studies have found a higher prevalence in women compared to men (Sakakibara et al., 2001). Patients with more advanced PD are more likely to report nocturia (Barone et al., 2009). A small study of 23 PD patients with nocturia reported a frequency of nocturnal micturition episodes ranging from 1 to 7/night, with a mean of 3.5 (Smith et al., 2015).

Nocturia is the most common lower urinary tract symptom in PD (Campos-Sousa et al., 2003), but is often comorbid with other lower urinary tract symptoms including daytime urinary frequency, urgency, and incomplete bladder emptying. As mentioned, in some patients with nocturia, polyuria is present: the passing of large (excessive) amounts. In one small study of 23 PD patients with nocturia (Smith et al., 2015), polyuria was seen in 13 (56%), and was associated with worse subject sleep quality.

Some patients have difficulty distinguishing between sleep fragmentation resulting from nocturia versus "convenience voiding," which is urination that occurs when the patient is awakened for other reasons (not by the need to urinate).

Etiology and differential diagnosis

Several different causes of and contributors to nocturia occur in PD. Etiologies unrelated to PD must be considered including but not limited to obstructive sleep apnea, congestive heart failure, and diabetes. Urologic evaluation to evaluate for structural etiologies, such as benign prostatic hypertrophy or bladder calculi, is indicated. Tests that may aid in diagnosis include ultrasound to examine postvoid residual volume, and urodynamic studies. In select cases, especially where obstruction is suspected, cystoscopy may be necessary. Several medications can also contribute to nocturia and the patient's medication list should be reviewed carefully. In patients with acute urinary symptoms evaluation for infection with urine analysis is indicated.

Having the patient keep a bladder diary is critical to diagnosing nocturia, distinguishing it from mimics, and identifying contributors to it. The diary should document not only number and time of nighttime urination episodes but also urine volume. This is critical in distinguishing in determining whether polyuria is present.

What few data are available from urodynamic studies published on patients with PD indicate that in most patients with PD, nocturia likely results from neurogenic detrusor overactivity (Ragab & Mohammed, 2011; Uchiyama et al., 2011; Xue, Wang, Zong, & Zhang, 2014). This in turn may result from loss of inhibition of the central micturition center, with consequent disinhibition of the micturition reflex. Reduced functional bladder capacity at night and incomplete bladder emptying are other significant contributors (Batla et al., 2016). Although some patients have elevated frequency of urination overnight, the volume of urine output may not be dramatic. Anecdotally, this may especially be the case in patients with anxiety that contributes to presleep urinary frequency, sleep initiation insomnia, and even nocturia. However, as mentioned earlier, nocturnal polyuria may occur in many patients with nocturia. The pathophysiology of nocturnal polyuria may be mediated by abnormalities in secretion of antidiuretic hormone and atrial natriuretic peptide, which in turn may be secondary to abnormalities in the circadian rhythm in PD. See Chapter 9 for more on circadian dysfunction in PD.

Autonomic dysfunction in PD may also contribute to nocturia. Autonomic dysfunction may result in abnormalities in mineralocorticoid secretion. This in turn may lead to a lack of the normal reduction in blood pressure that occurs overnight, and/or even supine hypertension (even in those with daytime orthostatic hypotension). These nocturnal blood pressure abnormalities in turn may contribute to nocturia via increased release of atrial natriuretic peptide, among other mechanisms.

As for the effects of PD-specific medications on nocturia, there are little data available in this regard. Some findings regarding the effects of levodopa on urinary function in PD in general are worth considering. In interpreting studies on this, it is important to consider that it is possible there are differing acute and chronic effects of levodopa on bladder function, and on subjective urinary symptoms. In one study of 18 PD patients that included urodynamic studies pre- and post a 100 mg dose of levodopa, a worsening of detrusor hyperreflexia postdose was found (Uchiyama, Sakakibara, Hattori, & Yamanishi, 2003). On the other hand, in a study of 32 patients, urodynamic studies were performed on patients who were on chronic, stable regimens of dopaminergic medications and then again after medications were withdrawn (Winge, Werdelin, Nielsen, & Stimpel, 2004). Among those with subjective urinary symptoms, bladder capacity was higher in the medicated state. To specifically investigate acute versus chronic effects, one study of 26 levodopa-naïve PD patients with urinary urgency were studied (Brusa et al., 2007). Urodynamic studies were conducted before levodopa therapy, 1 hour after a 200 mg dose of levodopa, and then again 2 months after a stable levodopa regimen of a mean daily dose of 300 mg (± 150 mg). As in the study by Uchiyama et al. discussed earlier (Uchiyama et al., 2003), after acute administration of levodopa, there was worsening of bladder overactivity (neurogenic detrusor contractions) and bladder capacity. However, the urodynamic studies performed on the same patients 2 months after initiation of levo-dopa regimen demonstrated a 120% improvement in the amount of bladder volume required for first sensation bladder filling, a 93% improvement in neurogenic detrusor contractions, and a 33% improvement in bladder capacity (Brusa et al., 2007).

As for the differential diagnosis, nocturia is to be distinguished from nocturnal incontinence and enuresis. Although both of these may be comorbid with nocturia, their causes and even treatments may differ, and thus distinction between them is important. Nocturnal incontinence is just as the name implies: incontinence occurring at night. The causes to nocturnal incontinence in PD are many. Some patients report nocturnal incontinence results from motor symptoms precluding them from getting to the bathroom in the required time. In other patients with cognitive dysfunction/dementia, there may be an inability to recognize and communicate (to caregivers) the need to urinate in a timely manner. Overflow incontinence from bladder outlet obstruction is also one etiology. On the other hand, enuresis is defined as incontinence that occurs during sleep.

Consequences and complications

Nocturia adversely affects quality of life in PD (Martinez-Martin, Rodriguez-Blazquez, Kurtis, Chaudhuri, & NMSS Validation Group, 2011). Nocturia is a major contributor to poor subjective sleep quality, and it influences objective sleep as well. In regards to the latter, it is associated with lower total sleep time and sleep efficiency (Vaughan, Juncos, Trotti, Johnson, & Bliwise, 2013). In addition, it is associated with increased risk of falls (Balash et al., 2005), and extrapolating from data in the general older adult population, may be associated with increased risk of hip fracture as well (Asplund, 2006). Another important consequence of nocturia in PD is that it adversely affects caregiver sleep as well (Batla et al., 2016).

Management

The management of nocturia in PD is multipronged and requires multidisciplinary effort along with input from the patient's neurologist, the patient's primary care provider, and possibly a urologist (Table 10.1).

A close examination of the patient's medication list is critical when attempting to reduce the frequency of nocturia. Where diuretics are necessary for comorbid medical conditions, they should be dosed in the morning, and long-acting diuretics should be avoided. Restriction of evening water intake should be advised. Pilot data indicate that pelvic floor exercises may be useful in treating lower urinary tract symptoms, including nocturia, in PD. In a small 8-week study in 17 patients of an exercise-based, biofeedback-assisted behavioral intervention (Vaughan et al., 2011), participants received instruction and training on pelvic floor muscle exercises (facilitated by computer-assisted EMG biofeedback), and bladder control strategies including

Table 10.1 Management options for nocturia in PD.

Category	Treatment	Comment
Behavioral	Minimize intake of liquids in the afternoon/evening	This recommendation should be accompanied by counseling for adequate daytime hydration especially in patients with orthostatic hypotension
	Limit caffeine intake especially in the afternoon/evening	This would be particularly important in patients with multifactorial insomnia
	Timed urination before bed	
	Consider equipment to minimize risk of nighttime falls	Urinal, bedside commode, external (condom) catheter
Rehabilitation	Pelvic floor exercises	
Medications	Withdrawal of medications that can contribute to nocturia	If the patient requires diuretics, their dosing in the morning, and avoidance of long-acting diuretics, is required
	PD medications	Optimize overnight motor symptom control
	Anticholinergics	Anticholinergic with the least binding to central muscarinic receptors should be used, and avoided all together in patients with cognitive dysfunction/dementia
	β-Agonist	Mirabegron likely has a lower risk side-effect profile as compared to anticholinergics in PD (based on extrapolation of data from the general older adult population)
	α-Blockers	α-Blockers may be recommended in select cases by urologists where bladder outlet obstruction due to prostate enlargement or other structural causes are present. However, there is a high risk of orthostatic hypotension that may limit or even contraindicate use of these agents in PD
	Desmopressin	Desmopressin treats polyuria that is often comorbid with nocturia in PD and may cause or contribute to it. Limited data indicate a high risk of hyponatremia in older adults, and desmopressin should be used with extreme caution in PD, especially in those aged over 65.

Continued

Table 10.1 Management options for nocturia in PD.—*cont'd*

Category	Treatment	Comment
Chemodenervation	Botulinum toxin injection into detrusor muscle	Detrusor botulinum toxin injection (administered by trained urologists) could be considered in select PD patients. However, the patient should be counseled that an adverse event that may occur is urinary retention requiring intermittent catheterization.

urge suppression. Self-reported (questionnaire-assessed) frequency of urinary urgency and incontinence improved, and there was a trend toward improvement in nocturia as well.

In patients in whom interventions do not eliminate nocturia, instituting safety measures to reduce risk of falls and/or other injuries when the patient gets up to go to the bathroom at night is critical. The path to the bathroom should be well lit. When possible/necessary, eliminating the need to get to the bathroom for urination may be achieved with a bedside portable commode, and/or use of urinals. For patients who have comorbid nocturnal incontinence, use of adult diapers can help reduce patient distress and caregiver burden. In men, a "condom catheter" may be useful to this effect as well. Optimizing motor symptom control is also necessary to help with the mobility required to get to the bathroom safely. Consideration for bedtime dosing of controlled-release levodopa, and/or prescription of inhaled levodopa (LeWitt et al., 2016), is indicated. Of note, deep brain stimulation surgery, a treatment for advanced PD, may help to improve lower urinary tract symptoms, including nocturia, as well (Winge & Nielsen, 2012).

Pharmacotherapy for lower urinary tract symptoms in PD is often necessary and may help with nocturia (Table 10.1). Evidence to support these treatments for nocturia in PD is limited, and recommendations are derived from small studies in PD and from data from the general older adult population. Anticholinergic agents are the mainstay of therapy as they target neurogenic detrusor overactivity, a key contributor to nocturia. In the Movement Disorders Society evidence-based review on treatments of nonmotor symptoms of PD (Seppi et al., 2019), solifenacin was considered to have insufficient evidence and to be possibly useful for treatment of lower urinary tract symptoms (though not specifically nocturia). However, use of anticholinergic agents carries risk of important side effects that can be detrimental in PD. These range from peripheral side effects such as constipation to central side effects such as confusion and hallucinations, especially in those with cognitive dysfunction. Thus, where possible, use of agents with least penetrance of the blood brain barrier/least likelihood of action at central muscarinic receptors is strongly recommended (Chancellor & Boone, 2012). For example, oxybutynin is most likely to cross the blood brain barrier and to have action at multiple muscarinic receptors. Tolterodine, solifenacin, and darifenacin have lower CNS penetrance as compared to oxybutynin; trospium and fesoterodine have the least CNS penetration and are associated with the least risk of central nervous system side effects (Chancellor & Boone, 2012). Use of other drug classes to treat detrusor overactivity, such as mirabegron, may be indicated though again guided by limited evidence for safety and efficacy in PD (Peyronnet et al., 2018). Studies from the general older adult population indicate that desmopressin improves polyuria (Mattiasson, Abrams, Van Kerrebroeck, Walter, & Weiss, 2002) but it carries a risk of hyponatremia especially in older adults, and should only be used in select PD cases while exercising caution and close monitoring. In select cases, chemodenervation of the bladder with botulinum toxin may be considered (Giannantoni et al., 2009), especially in cases with quality-of-life-limiting daytime urinary symptoms as well.

Illustrative case in context

In the case described, the patient has frequent nighttime urination and the history also indicates that he has polyuria (as he is reporting similar output of urine volume during micturition episodes at night as compared to daytime micturition episodes). This is disrupting his sleep, and leading to daytime tiredness. The initial approach should be to have him keep an overnight bladder diary. A thorough review of his medication list, especially for evening diuretic dosing, should also occur. He should be counseled on avoiding liquids in the afternoons/evenings, as well as caffeine. Referral to a urologist is indicated to rule out benign prostatic hypertrophy or other structural problems. If the determination is neurogenic detrusor overactivity (which is the most likely cause or at least a big contributor), consideration for pharmacotherapy is indicated. Given his age, a medication for overactive bladder that does not have high risk of central cholinergic side effects should be selected. Mirabegron, trospium, and/or fesoterodine would be good considerations for him. A thorough sleep history should be obtained and if concern for sleep apnea arises, and/or if he does not respond to medications for overactive bladder, a polysomnogram would be appropriate, as obstructive sleep apnea can cause or contribute to nocturia. Finally, if he continues to be troubled by so many episodes of nocturia despite optimal medical therapy, bladder chemodenervation could be considered in consultation with a urologist, but keeping in mind there is a risk of urinary retention requiring intermittent self-catheterization.

References

Asplund, R. (2006). Hip fractures, nocturia, and nocturnal polyuria in the elderly. *Archives of Gerontology and Geriatrics, 43*(3), 319−326.

Balash, Y., Peretz, C., Leibovich, G., Herman, T., Hausdorff, J. M., & Giladi, N. (2005). Falls in outpatients with Parkinson's disease: Frequency, impact and identifying factors. *Journal of Neurology, 252*(11), 1310−1315.

Barone, P., Antonini, A., Colosimo, C., Marconi, R., Morgante, L., Avarello, T. P., et al. (2009). The PRIAMO study: A multicenter assessment of nonmotor symptoms and their impact on quality of life in Parkinson's disease. *Movement Disorders: Official Journal of the Movement Disorder Society, 24*(11), 1641−1649.

Batla, A., Phe, V., De Min, L., & Panicker, J. N. (2016). Nocturia in Parkinson's disease: Why does it occur and how to manage? *Movement Disorders Clinical Practice, 3*(5), 443−451.

Brusa, L., Petta, F., Pisani, A., Moschella, V., Iani, C., Stanzione, P., et al. (2007). Acute vs chronic effects of l-dopa on bladder function in patients with mild Parkinson disease. *Neurology, 68*(18), 1455−1459.

Campos-Sousa, R. N., Quagliato, E., da Silva, B. B., de Carvalho, R. M., Jr., Ribeiro, S. C., & de Carvalho, D. F. (2003). Urinary symptoms in Parkinson's disease: Prevalence and associated factors. *Arquivos de Neuro-Psiquiatria, 61*(2B), 359−363.

Chancellor, M., & Boone, T. (2012). Anticholinergics for overactive bladder therapy: Central nervous system effects. *CNS Neuroscience and Therapeutics, 18*(2), 167−174.

Giannantoni, A., Rossi, A., Mearini, E., Del Zingaro, M., Porena, M., & Berardelli, A. (2009). Botulinum toxin A for overactive bladder and detrusor muscle overactivity in patients with Parkinson's disease and multiple system atrophy. *The Journal of Urology, 182*(4), 1453−1457.

Hashim, H., Blanker, M. H., Drake, M. J., Djurhuus, J. C., Meijlink, J., Morris, V., et al. (2019). International Continence Society (ICS) report on the terminology for nocturia and nocturnal lower urinary tract function. *Neurourology and Urodynamics, 38*(2), 499−508.

LeWitt, P. A., Hauser, R. A., Grosset, D. G., Stocchi, F., Saint-Hilaire, M. H., Ellenbogen, A., et al. (2016). A randomized trial of inhaled levodopa (CVT-301) for motor fluctuations in Parkinson's disease. *Movement Disorders: Official Journal of the Movement Disorder Society, 31*(9), 1356−1365.

Martinez-Martin, P., Rodriguez-Blazquez, C., Kurtis, M. M., Chaudhuri, K. R., & NMSS Validation Group. (2011). The impact of non-motor symptoms on health-related quality of life of patients with Parkinson's disease. *Movement Disorders: Official Journal of the Movement Disorder Society, 26*(3), 399−406.

Mattiasson, A., Abrams, P., Van Kerrebroeck, P., Walter, S., & Weiss, J. (2002). Efficacy of desmopressin in the treatment of nocturia: A double-blind placebo-controlled study in men. *BJU International, 89*(9), 855−862.

Peyronnet, B., Vurture, G., Palma, J. A., Malacarne, D. R., Feigin, A., Sussman, R. D., et al. (2018). Mirabegron in patients with Parkinson disease and overactive bladder symptoms: A retrospective cohort. *Parkinsonism & Related Disorders, 57*, 22−26.

Ragab, M. M., & Mohammed, E. S. (2011). Idiopathic Parkinson's disease patients at the urologic clinic. *Neurourology and Urodynamics, 30*(7), 1258−1261.

Sakakibara, R., Shinotoh, H., Uchiyama, T., Sakuma, M., Kashiwado, M., Yoshiyama, M., et al. (2001). Questionnaire-based assessment of pelvic organ dysfunction in Parkinson's disease. *Autonomic Neuroscience: Basic & Clinical, 92*(1−2), 76−85.

Sammour, Z. M., Gomes, C. M., Barbosa, E. R., Lopes, R. I., Sallem, F. S., Trigo-Rocha, F. E., et al. (2009). Voiding dysfunction in patients with Parkinson's disease: Impact of neurological impairment and clinical parameters. *Neurourology and Urodynamics, 28*(6), 510−515.

Seppi, K., Ray Chaudhuri, K., Coelho, M., Fox, S. H., Katzenschlager, R., Perez Lloret, S., et al. (2019). Update on treatments for nonmotor symptoms of Parkinson's disease-an evidence-based medicine review. *Movement Disorders: Official Journal of the Movement Disorder Society, 34*(2), 180−198.

Smith, M., Seth, J., Batla, A., Hofereiter, J., Bhatia, K. P., & Panicker, J. N. (2015). Nocturia in patients with Parkinson's disease. *Movement Disorders Clinical Practice, 3*(2), 168−172.

Uchiyama, T., Sakakibara, R., Hattori, T., & Yamanishi, T. (2003). Short-term effect of a single levodopa dose on micturition disturbance in Parkinson's disease patients with the wearing-off phenomenon. *Movement Disorders: Official Journal of the Movement Disorder Society, 18*(5), 573−578.

Uchiyama, T., Sakakibara, R., Yamamoto, T., Ito, T., Yamaguchi, C., Awa, Y., et al. (2011). Urinary dysfunction in early and untreated Parkinson's disease. *Journal of Neurology, Neurosurgery & Psychiatry, 82*(12), 1382−1386.

Vaughan, C. P., Juncos, J. L., Burgio, K. L., Goode, P. S., Wolf, R. A., & Johnson, T. M., 2nd (2011). Behavioral therapy to treat urinary incontinence in Parkinson disease. *Neurology, 76*(19), 1631−1634.

Vaughan, C. P., Juncos, J. L., Trotti, L. M., Johnson, T. M., 2nd, & Bliwise, D. L. (2013). Nocturia and overnight polysomnography in Parkinson disease. *Neurourology and Urodynamics, 32*(8), 1080−1085.

Winge, K., & Nielsen, K. K. (2012). Bladder dysfunction in advanced Parkinson's disease. *Neurourology and Urodynamics, 31*(8), 1279−1283.

Winge, K., Skau, A. M., Stimpel, H., Nielsen, K. K., & Werdelin, L. (2006). Prevalence of bladder dysfunction in Parkinsons disease. *Neurourology and Urodynamics, 25*(2), 116−122.

Winge, K., Werdelin, L. M., Nielsen, K. K., & Stimpel, H. (2004). Effects of dopaminergic treatment on bladder function in Parkinson's disease. *Neurourology and Urodynamics, 23*(7), 689−696.

Xue, P., Wang, T., Zong, H., & Zhang, Y. (2014). Urodynamic analysis and treatment of male Parkinson's disease patients with voiding dysfunction. *Chinese Medical Journal, 127*(5), 878−881.

Sleep benefit

Illustrative case

A 62-year-old man has had Parkinson's disease (PD) for 11 years. On a typical day, he has motor fluctuations, marked by "OFF" periods in which he suffers stiffness, slowness of movement, and tremor, and "ON" periods, usually occurring about 45 minutes after a dose of levodopa (200 mg), whereby his symptoms are well controlled and he has only minimal tremor, but sometimes also has dyskinesias, especially later on in the day. He does report that sometimes, upon awakening from sleep, he will find himself to be free of PD symptoms, the way he feels when he is "ON" (medicated), despite not having taken a levodopa dose in the preceding several hours (sometimes up to 8 hours, depending on how long he had slept overnight). This feeling of being free of motor symptoms upon awakening, when it occurs, may last for up to 1 hour. This does not happen on all nights, but when it does happen, he often delays intake of his first dose of levodopa until his motor symptoms emerge. He does not feel as though this delay has adverse consequences, and feels the advantage to this is that it helps reduce the probability that he will have bothersome dyskinesias later on in the day.

Overview
Definition

Sleep benefit is the phenomenon observed in some patients with PD, whereby their motor symptoms are transiently under control upon awakening. This is observed despite them not having taken PD medications for several hours. Although the degree of control of symptoms varies (van Gilst, Bloem, & Overeem, 2013), some PD patients describe absence or near absence of motor symptoms on awakening; some patients (about one-fifth) even describe the sleep benefit exceeding motor control as compared to maximal medication effect (van Gilst, Bloem et al., 2015). Indeed, in some studies, the more conservative definition of sleep benefit is specific to the feeling of being "ON" (i.e., feeling as good as the patient typically feels after

Disorders of Sleep and Wakefulness in Parkinson's Disease. https://doi.org/10.1016/B978-0-323-67374-7.00011-0

having taken PD medication and it having maximal benefit): "the experience of a temporary decrease in PD symptoms upon awakening after a period of sleep (night or daytime) before drug intake; the patient is feeling as good as "on" (or better)" (van Gilst, Bloem et al., 2015).

Sleep benefit is typically reported in the context of awakening in the morning after nighttime sleep, but can also occur after daytime naps (Merello et al., 1997; van Gilst et al., 2013; van Gilst, Louter, Baumann, Bloem, & Overeem, 2012). This period of motor control following sleep typically lasts for about 1 hour (though the range is as little as 3 minutes to as long as 5 hours) (van Gilst et al., 2013; van Gilst, Bloem et al., 2015).

Epidemiology

Data on the epidemiology of sleep benefit in PD are limited, and vary according to the definition of sleep benefit used (van Gilst et al., 2013), and whether sleep benefit was defined based on examination of the patient by an experienced rater upon awakening, via patient interview (Currie, Bennett, Harrison, Trugman, & Wooten, 1997), via survey about sleep benefit, or via survey about motor symptoms or function in the morning (van Gilst, Bloem et al., 2015).

In one of the first systematic studies of sleep benefit in PD, 16 PD patients were observed as part of an inpatient study (Bateman, Levett, & Marsden, 1999). Motor examinations were administered in the morning, immediately upon the subjects awakening from sleep. Sleep benefit was observed in 6 (38%). Moreover, 113 PD patients were then administered a questionnaire to investigate their subjective report of sleep benefit (Bateman et al., 1999). Participants were also asked to complete activities of daily living questionnaire three times in 1 day: once immediately upon awakening, before taking any medications, once after taking medications and when they felt their medications were working at their best (typical "ON" state), and once when their medications had worn off and were without any effect (maximal "OFF" state). In addition, 66 (58.4%) reported a subjective sleep benefit and 49 (43%) had a change in the activities of daily living score of 12 or more which was deemed consistent with evidence of sleep benefit. Participants estimated the sleep benefit to last from 10 to >150 minutes; mean 87 minutes. Younger patients were more likely to report sleep benefit (Bateman et al., 1999).

Another study assessed for sleep benefit via interview of 162 PD patients presenting to an outpatient Movement Disorders clinic (Currie et al., 1997). Among them, 53 (33%) reported sleep benefit.

In one of the largest survey studies of sleep benefit after nighttime and daytime sleep in PD, 253 PD patients were administered a questionnaire that defined sleep benefit as a "clear decrease in PD symptoms after a period of sleep" (van Gilst et al., 2012). Participants also completed a range of nonmotor assessments including a subjective sleep quality scale, the Pittsburgh Sleep Quality Index (PSQI), and the Epworth Sleepiness Scale to measure daytime sleepiness. Among the final sample of 243 who completed the survey, 114 (46.9%) indicated that they experience sleep benefit. Of those, 33 (13.8%) also reported sleep benefit after daytime naps. Interestingly, 13 (13.3%) reported sleep benefit only after daytime sleep, but not nighttime sleep. The PSQI did not differ in those two latter groups (van Gilst et al., 2012).

Of note, not all patients with sleep benefit experience it after each period of sleep. Indeed, in a prospective questionnaire-based study, none of the patients with sleep benefit reported sleep benefit 7 nights/week (van Gilst, Bloem et al., 2015). Rather, most patients with sleep benefit reported experiencing it 1−3 nights a week, with a minority experiencing it 4, 5, or 6 nights a week (van Gilst, Bloem et al., 2015).

To summarize, sleep benefit in PD, when determined via examination, is present in about 40% (Bateman et al., 1999) of patients and reported subjectively by survey or interview in about 33%−60% (mean 44%) (Bateman et al., 1999; Currie et al., 1997; Merello et al., 1997; van Gilst et al., 2012, 2013). Several studies, including a meta-analysis of seven papers, demonstrate that sleep benefit is more common in those with longer disease duration (Bateman et al., 1999; Currie et al., 1997; Rui, Qingling, Xinyue, Xin, & Weihong, 2019; van Gilst et al., 2013; van Gilst, Bloem et al., 2015). The meta-analysis also found sleep benefit to be related to more severe PD disease severity (as measured with physical exam−based motor score, the Movement Disorders Society Unified Parkinson's Disease Rating Scale Part III). Limited data indicate that sleep benefit is also more likely in those with daytime motor fluctuations (Bateman et al., 1999). PD patients with sleep benefit report higher doses of levodopa therapy (Currie et al., 1997) and longer durations of levodopa exposure (Currie et al., 1997; van Gilst, Bloem et al., 2015).

Data also indicate that sleep benefit may be more likely with younger ages of PD onset (Bateman et al., 1999; Currie et al., 1997; van Gilst et al., 2013; van Gilst, Bloem et al., 2015); the meta-analysis did not confirm this but that meta-analysis did find significant heterogeneity in studies (Rui et al., 2019). One study found a male predominance (Merello et al., 1997) though this has not been shown in other studies that assessed for sleep benefit (Currie et al., 1997; Rui et al., 2019; van Gilst et al., 2013; van Gilst, Bloem et al., 2015).

Etiology and differential diagnosis

The etiology of sleep benefit in PD has not been elucidated, but several interesting hypotheses have been put forth.

One possible hypothesis to explain sleep benefit posits that it results from a direct physiologic effect of sleep to enhance dopaminergic storage and transmission (Bateman et al., 1999; Merello et al., 1997). However, there are few data in humans that support this possibility; in fact, some studies indicate worse sleep quality in those with sleep benefit. Animal studies are not conclusive in this regard, but do suggest a change in the temporal pattern of dopaminergic neuron firing during sleep in PD (Monti & Monti, 2007) and differential effects of sleep deprivation on D1, D2, and D3 receptor subtypes (Lim, Xu, Holtzman, & Mach, 2011).

In one of the few studies to objectively assess for sleep benefit, 20 PD patients were identified, 10 with sleep benefit and 10 without (Hogl et al., 1998). Presence or absence of sleep benefit was ascertained via questionnaire. Sleep benefit was defined as subjective "motor restoration" after a night's sleep, and a subjective improvement or resolution of PD symptoms lasting at least 1 hour. The comparator group without sleep benefit had to report worse motor function in the morning as compared to their function following PD medication intake. The two groups with and without sleep benefit were matched on age, gender, and disease duration. Motor examination was performed by a rater blinded to presence/absence of sleep benefit. It was conducted serially, at night before sleep and immediately upon spontaneous awakening, then every 30 minutes for about 1.5 hours. The subjects then took their usual levodopa dose and were subsequently examined until return to baseline motor state or worse. During this time, patients' subjective assessment of their motor function was also ascertained. Patients also completed questionnaires regarding activities of daily living, PD symptoms, depression, and circadian rhythm. Blood samples were obtained twice during basal morning state and after levodopa intake. In addition, overnight polysomnography was performed. The study found that the sleep benefit group had a mean −6.5 difference (improvement) in postsleep versus presleep motor score, where the group without sleep benefit had a mean +3.9 difference (worsening). Of note, though, objective motor scores were not necessarily congruent with patient's subjective assessment of their motor symptoms. After levodopa administration in the morning, both the sleep benefit group and the group without sleep benefit had a significant improvement in motor score, with no difference in magnitude of improvement between the groups. The rate of dyskinesias did not differ between the groups. As for the levodopa pharmacokinetic data, residual levodopa was not detected in the morning plasma samples in any patient. There were no differences in time to reach maximal levodopa concentration, or the concentration itself, between the sleep benefit versus no sleep benefit group (150 vs. 157 mg, respectively). Regarding the relationship between objective sleep measures and sleep benefit, sleep was abnormal in both groups, including low sleep efficiency, low amounts of rapid eye movement (REM) sleep, and a high number of arousals. There were no differences in REM without atonia, or history of dream enactment, in both groups (see Chapter 6 for more on REM without atonia). As for subjective sleep, patients rated their overall sleep quality similarly. Finally, a measure of circadian function, a "morningness—eveningness" questionnaire, found no differences in circadian type predominance between the groups. The small sample size in this study limits the conclusions that can be drawn from it, but it nevertheless sheds some insight to the potential explanations (or lack thereof) for sleep benefit in PD (Hogl et al., 1998).

In another approach to objectively measuring sleep benefit, 18 PD patients with subjective sleep benefit, 20 without sleep benefit, and 20 non-PD controls performed the timed pegboard dexterity task and quantified finger tapping task after an observed overnight sleep and/or nap (van Gilst, van Mierlo, Bloem, & Overeem, 2015). Overnight polysomnography was recorded. There were no differences between groups in total sleep time, sleep efficiency, or sleep stages. In addition, there were no differences in subjective sleep quality. As for postsleep versus presleep performance on the pegboard task, it was on average slower in the morning, but with no significant difference between the group with subjective sleep benefit versus those without. There was no significant difference in postsleep versus presleep in the finger tapping tasks and no difference between the groups with versus without sleep benefit either. Subjective motor measures (motor symptom diary responses) were also not different between the groups. The authors suggested that patients with sleep benefit may misperceive their motor symptoms on awakening, such that sleep benefit may be a subjective experience that does not translate clinically into objective motor improvement or function in all cases (van Gilst, van Mierlo et al., 2015). The same group found similar results in a study of 240 PD patients administered a diary of motor function and a questionnaire regarding sleep benefit (van Gilst, van Mierlo et al., 2015). Here too, they found that subjective experience of sleep benefit did not translate into improvement in motor function as reflected on the diary. To what degree the night-to-night variability in sleep benefit (van Gilst, van Mierlo et al., 2015) influences the discordance between perceived sleep benefit, objective sleep benefit, and motor function following sleep is not clear.

In yet another study that objectively measured sleep benefit following objectively-assessed sleep, 60 PD patients underwent polysomnography and 38 also underwent 2-week actigraphy (Sherif, Valko, Overeem, & Baumann, 2014). Total sleep time on polysomnography was shorter in those with sleep benefit compared to those without (272 vs. 346 minutes, respectively), and similar results were reflected in the actigraphy data (though nonsignificant). The sleep benefit group also had longer sleep latency compared to those without (81 vs. 26 minutes, respectively). Sleep architecture (time spent in different sleep stages) was not different between those with versus without sleep benefit. The authors indicated their data may argue against the hypothesis that sleep benefit results from direct or indirect beneficial effects of sleep on motor function. One possibility suggested is that better night time sleep could indicate an overall propensity toward sleeping/sleepiness that may in turn affect motor function via vigilance (Sherif et al., 2014). In contrast, as detailed earlier, two studies did not support the idea that sleep quality per se influences the manifestation of sleep benefit in either direction (Hogl et al., 1998; van Gilst, van Mierlo et al., 2015). Regarding the relationship between subjective sleep quality and sleep benefit, one study found that based on survey responses, PD patients who reported sleep benefit reported shorter sleep durations and lower sleep efficiency (van Gilst, van Mierlo et al., 2015). However, absolute differences were quite small, and this was not replicated in another study (van Gilst et al., 2012).

There are few data regarding the relationship between sleep benefit and PD medications. One study reported a higher daily dose of levodopa in those with sleep benefit compared to those without (Currie et al., 1997), but this has not been consistent across studies (van Gilst et al., 2012, 2013). PD patients with sleep benefit were also more likely to be on controlled-release formulations of levodopa compared to those without (Currie et al., 1997). It has been hypothesized that sleep benefit may result from higher residual morning plasma concentrations of levodopa; however, in a small study that sampled morning levodopa plasma levels and correlated them with motor examination, this was not supported (Hogl et al., 1998).

On the other hand, another possibility proposed is that sleep benefit is just within the realm of the phenomenon of motor fluctuations seen in some patients with PD with advancing disease, related to the time of day ("morning benefit") as opposed to the direct consequence of sleep (Factor & Weiner, 1998). However, the observation regarding sleep benefit following daytime naps brings this explanation into question (Merello et al., 1997; van Gilst et al., 2012, 2013), as does the higher self-reported prevalence of wearing off phenomena in PD patients without sleep benefit compared to those who report sleep benefit (Currie et al., 1997).

Sleep benefit does not seem to be related to several other nonmotor features seen in PD including depression (van Gilst et al., 2012), and daytime sleepiness (Sherif et al., 2014; van Gilst et al., 2012). Some reports have suggested that patients with PD due to *parkin* gene mutation may be particularly likely to experience sleep benefit (van Gilst et al., 2013).

Why some patients with PD awaken to find an improvement in symptoms and others awaken after a night's sleep with significant PD symptoms is not clear. The latter is seen in patients with morning akinesia, also called as early morning off (Rizos et al., 2014). PD patients with morning akinesia awaken in the OFF state: their PD motor and nonmotor symptoms are substantial, and such patients often cite their PD symptoms as being *worst* in the morning (in contrast to patients with sleep benefit who often feel best in the mornings). Morning akinesia is essentially a result of being unmedicated after a nightlong treatment-free period. In a multicenter survey study of 320 PD patients with mean disease duration of 7 years, it was identified in 60%. Morning akinesia/early morning off is associated with a significant negative impact on quality of life and increased caregiver burden (Onozawa et al., 2016; Viwattanakulvanid et al., 2014). In addition, many PD patients have delayed ON and/or suboptimal ON after their first dose of PD medications for the day: the time the first dose of the day of PD medications takes to take effect (to "kick in") is perceived by the patient as being prolonged (>30 minutes) and/or the benefit of that dose is less than usual/expected. In one survey study of 151 PD patients with advanced PD (as defined by presence of motor fluctuations), delayed ON/suboptimal ON was reported to occur at least once a week in about 60%, and every day in 20% (though it is of note that the estimated morning time-to-ON, as ascertained via patient diaries, was only a few minutes longer than time-to-ON for other doses of the day) (Stocchi, Coletti, Bonassi, Radicati, & Vacca, 2019). Evidence to guide management of morning akinesia/early morning off and delayed/suboptimal ON is limited. Some interventions that could be helpful include sustained release doses of levodopa taken at bedtime, overnight dosing of levodopa, long-acting dopamine agonists at bedtime (with the highest level of evidence available for rotigotine (LeWitt et al., 2013; Trenkwalder et al., 2011; 2012)), subcutaneous apomorphine (LeWitt, Ondo, Van Lunen, & Bottini, 2009), and inhaled levodopa (LeWitt et al., 2016). An understanding of sleep benefit could translate into improved treatments for patients with morning akinesia/early morning OFF periods and delayed ON periods.

Consequences and complications

Some PD patients with sleep benefit report the mornings to be their best time of day (Merello et al., 1997). Patients with sleep benefit may be able to delay their first dose of PD medications, in the morning or when daytime napping leads to sleep benefit, or they may be able to skip their dose all together after sleep. Thus, there seem to be theoretical advantages to understanding sleep benefit such that the mechanisms that underlie it can be capitalized on to develop therapies that improve motor function in PD.

Management

In select patients who report sleep benefit, it is reasonable for them to delay their first dose of PD medication until the subjective sleep benefit has worn off, as long as delaying that dose does not seem to be associated with worse-than-usual motor symptoms (due to, for example, extending the period without medication) once the sleep benefit resolves.

Illustrative case in context

In the case described, the patient has advanced PD with motor fluctuations. The description is typical of sleep benefit, and it is not unreasonable for him to skip his first dose of PD medications on mornings he has sleep benefit, especially because he has found this reduces dyskinesias on days he is able to do so.

References

Bateman, D. E., Levett, K., & Marsden, C. D. (1999). Sleep benefit in Parkinson's disease. *Journal of Neurology, Neurosurgery & Psychiatry, 67*(3), 384–385.

Currie, L. J., Bennett, J. P., Jr., Harrison, M. B., Trugman, J. M., & Wooten, G. F. (1997). Clinical correlates of sleep benefit in Parkinson's disease. *Neurology, 48*(4), 1115–1117.

Factor, S. A., & Weiner, W. J. (1998). Sleep benefit' in Parkinson's disease. *Neurology, 50*(5), 1514–1515.

van Gilst, M. M., Bloem, B. R., & Overeem, S. (2013). "Sleep benefit" in Parkinson's disease: A systematic review. *Parkinsonism & Related Disorders, 19*(7), 654–659.

van Gilst, M. M., Bloem, B. R., & Overeem, S. (2015). Prospective assessment of subjective sleep benefit in Parkinson's disease. *BMC Neurology, 15*, 2-014-0256-2.

van Gilst, M. M., Louter, M., Baumann, C. R., Bloem, B. R., & Overeem, S. (2012). Sleep benefit in Parkinson's disease: Time to revive an enigma? *Journal of Parkinson's Disease, 2*(2), 167–170.

van Gilst, M. M., van Mierlo, P., Bloem, B. R., & Overeem, S. (2015). Quantitative motor performance and sleep benefit in Parkinson disease. *Sleep, 38*(10), 1567–1573.

Hogl, B. E., Gomez-Arevalo, G., Garcia, S., Scipioni, O., Rubio, M., Blanco, M., et al. (1998). A clinical, pharmacologic, and polysomnographic study of sleep benefit in Parkinson's disease. *Neurology, 50*(5), 1332–1339.

LeWitt, P. A., Boroojerdi, B., Surmann, E., Poewe, W., & SP716 Study Group, & SP715 Study Group. (2013). Rotigotine transdermal system for long-term treatment of patients with advanced Parkinson's disease: Results of two open-label extension studies, CLEOPATRA-PD and PREFER. *Journal of Neural Transmission, 120*(7), 1069–1081.

LeWitt, P. A., Hauser, R. A., Grosset, D. G., Stocchi, F., Saint-Hilaire, M. H., Ellenbogen, A., et al. (2016). A randomized trial of inhaled levodopa (CVT-301) for motor fluctuations in Parkinson's disease. *Movement Disorders: Official Journal of the Movement Disorder Society, 31*(9), 1356–1365.

LeWitt, P. A., Ondo, W. G., Van Lunen, B., & Bottini, P. B. (2009). Open-label study assessment of safety and adverse effects of subcutaneous apomorphine injections in treating "off" episodes in advanced Parkinson disease. *Clinical Neuropharmacology, 32*(2), 89–93.

Lim, M. M., Xu, J., Holtzman, D. M., & Mach, R. H. (2011). Sleep deprivation differentially affects dopamine receptor subtypes in mouse striatum. *NeuroReport, 22*(10), 489–493.

Merello, M., Hughes, A., Colosimo, C., Hoffman, M., Starkstein, S., & Leiguarda, R. (1997). Sleep benefit in Parkinson's disease. *Movement Disorders: Official Journal of the Movement Disorder Society, 12*(4), 506–508.

Monti, J. M., & Monti, D. (2007). The involvement of dopamine in the modulation of sleep and waking. *Sleep Medicine Reviews, 11*(2), 113–133.

Onozawa, R., Tsugawa, J., Tsuboi, Y., Fukae, J., Mishima, T., & Fujioka, S. (2016). The impact of early morning off in Parkinson's disease on patient quality of life and caregiver burden. *Journal of the Neurological Sciences, 364*, 1–5.

Rizos, A., Martinez-Martin, P., Odin, P., Antonini, A., Kessel, B., Kozul, T. K., et al. (2014). Characterizing motor and non-motor aspects of early-morning off periods in Parkinson's disease: An international multicenter study. *Parkinsonism & Related Disorders, 20*(11), 1231–1235.

Rui, Z., Qingling, C., Xinyue, Z., Xin, Z., & Weihong, L. (2019). The related factors of sleep benefit in Parkinson's disease: A systematic review and meta-analysis. *PLoS One, 14*(3), e0212951.

Sherif, E., Valko, P. O., Overeem, S., & Baumann, C. R. (2014). Sleep benefit in Parkinson's disease is associated with short sleep times. *Parkinsonism & Related Disorders, 20*(1), 116–118.

Stocchi, F., Coletti, C., Bonassi, S., Radicati, F. G., & Vacca, L. (2019). Early-morning OFF and levodopa dose failures in patients with Parkinson's disease attending a routine clinical appointment using Time-to-ON Questionnaire. *European Journal of Neurology, 26*(5), 821–826.

Trenkwaldera, C., Kiesb, B., Dioszeghyc, P., Hilld, D., Surmanne, E., Boroojerdie, B., et al. (2012). Rotigotine transdermal system for the management of motor function and sleep disturbances in Parkinson's disease: Results from a 1-year, open-label extension of the RECOVER study. *Basal Ganglia, 2*(2), 79–85.

Trenkwalder, C., Kies, B., Rudzinska, M., Fine, J., Nikl, J., Honczarenko, K., et al. (2011). Rotigotine effects on early morning motor function and sleep in Parkinson's disease: A double-blind, randomized, placebo-controlled study (RECOVER). *Movement Disorders: Official Journal of the Movement Disorder Society, 26*(1), 90–99.

Viwattanakulvanid, P., Kaewwilai, L., Jitkritsadakul, O., Brenden, N. R., Setthawatcharawanich, S., Boonrod, N., et al. (2014). The impact of the nocturnal disabilities of Parkinson's disease on caregivers' burden: Implications for interventions. *Journal of Neural Transmission, 121*(Suppl. 1), S15–S24.

Excessive daytime sleepiness

Illustrative Case—1

A 67-year-old man with Parkinson's disease (PD) presents accompanied by his wife for follow-up of PD. He reports being more sleepy lately. His wife confirms that he seems to doze off unintentionally, a lot more than he used to. For the past several years, he has fallen asleep everyday sitting in his recliner in the afternoon while reading or watching TV. However, in the preceding few months he had even fallen asleep a few times during meals or when sitting among company. He reports sleeping from 10 to 8 p.m., with good sleep quality aside from two to three brief episodes of awakening overnight. He does endorse feeling sleepy even soon after waking up. His wife does hear him snoring lightly sometimes. He denies depression.

His medication regimen includes levodopa 200 mg three times a day and extended-release pramipexole 1.5 mg. His motor symptoms are well controlled on this regimen.

Overview
Definition

Excessive daytime sleepiness in PD is classified under the "disorders of central hypersomnolence" according to the International Classification of Sleep Disorders (ICSD, third edition). Excessive daytime sleepiness, or hypersomnolence, is generally defined by the ICSD as "daily periods of irrepressible need to sleep or daytime lapses into sleep" (American Academy of Sleep Medicine, 2014).

Excessive daytime sleepiness (EDS) in PD is typically defined clinically based on a history of excessive and/or unintentional daytime sleepiness with frequent napping, whether intentional or unintentional. There are several questionnaires that measure daytime sleepiness that have been validated in PD including the Epworth Sleepiness Scale (ESS) (Hagell & Broman, 2007; Johns, 1991) and the scales for outcomes in Parkinson's disease-SLEEP-daytime sleepiness (SCOPA-SLEEP-DS) (Marinus, Visser, van Hilten, Lammers, & Stiggelbout, 2003). The Parkinson's Disease Sleep Scale (PDSS), PDSS2, and the Movement Disorders Society Unified

Disorders of Sleep and Wakefulness in Parkinson's Disease. https://doi.org/10.1016/B978-0-323-67374-7.00012-2

Parkinsons Disease Rating Scale (MDS-UPDRS) (Goetz et al., 2008) also have questions that ask about daytime sleepiness. There are two objective measures of hypersomnolence. The multiples sleep latency test (MSLT) measures propensity to fall asleep over five nap opportunities (American Academy of Sleep Medicine, 2014). The maintenance of wakefulness test (MWT), on the other hand, measures ability to stay awake over four trials (Littner et al., 2005). According to the ICSD3 (American Academy of Sleep Medicine, 2014), the objective finding on MSLT in patients with disorders of central hypersomnolence is mean sleep latency of eight or less minutes, with no more than 1 sleep-onset rapid eye movement (REM) period.

Epidemiology

Data on the prevalence of EDS in PD are largely based on use of interview or use of questionnaires for case ascertainment. EDS is significantly more likely to occur in PD compared to non-PD controls, even after adjusting for other factors such as age (Chotinaiwattarakul, Dayalu, Chervin, & Albin, 2011; Ferreira et al., 2006; Goulart et al., 2009; Knipe, Wickremaratchi, Wyatt-Haines, Morris, & Ben-Shlomo, 2011; Stavitsky, Saurman, McNamara, & Cronin-Golomb, 2010), though this may not be the case in early PD (Simuni et al., 2015).

In early PD, the prevalence of EDS based on ESS was 15%. Prevalence rate as high as 60%−70% have been reported in more advanced cohorts (Adler et al., 2011; Ataide, Franco, & Lins, 2014; Bjornara, Dietrichs, & Toft, 2014; Boddy et al., 2007; Borek, Kohn, & Friedman, 2006; Breen, Williams-Gray, Mason, Foltynie, & Barker, 2013; Chotinaiwattarakul et al., 2011; Cochen De Cock et al., 2014; Ferreira et al., 2006; Ferreira, Prabhakar, & Kharbanda, 2014; Gama et al., 2010; Gerbin, Viner, & Louis, 2012; Ghorayeb et al., 2007; Gjerstad, Alves, Wentzel-Larsen, Aarsland, & Larsen, 2006; Goulart et al., 2009; Happe, Baier, Bachmann, Helmschmied, & Paulus, 2008; Havlikova et al., 2011; Hu et al., 2011; Jongwanasiri, Prayoonwiwat, Pisarnpong, Srivanitchapoom, & Chotinaiwattarakul, 2014; Knipe et al., 2011; Larsson, Aarsland, Ballard, Minthon, & Londos, 2010; Louter et al., 2013; Monaca et al., 2006; Moreno-Lopez et al., 2011; Poryazova, Benninger, Waldvogel, & Bassetti, 2010; Prudon, Duncan, Khoo, Yarnall, & Anderson, 2014; Setthawatcharawanich, Limapichat, Sathirapanya, & Phabphal, 2011; Suzuki et al., 2008; Valko et al., 2010; Verbaan, van Rooden, Visser, Marinus, & van Hilten, 2008; Videnovic et al., 2014; Wang et al., 2010; Weerkamp et al., 2013; Yong, Fook-Chong, Pavanni, Lim, & Tan, 2011), such as nursing home residents (Weerkamp et al., 2013).

EDS is more likely in older patients with longer disease duration and greater disease severity (Gjerstad et al., 2006; Suzuki et al., 2007). Although it is often caused or exacerbated by PD medications, EDS can occur and progress independent of PD medications (Amara et al., 2017; Dhawan et al., 2006; Gjerstad et al., 2006). EDS is more likely in male PD patients compared to females (Ghorayeb et al., 2007; Gjerstad et al., 2006), even after adjusting for dopaminergic medication dose (Stavitsky & Cronin-Golomb, 2011). EDS may even precede the diagnosis of

PD, suggesting it may be a prodromal manifestation of the disease (Abbott et al., 2005).

In an incident cohort of 126 PD patients thought to be representative of the general PD population (Breen et al., 2013), EDS was assessed with ESS at baseline and follow-up. ESS was available at the 3.5-year follow-up assessment on 118 patients and 49% had EDS as defined by ESS >10. At the 5-year follow-up period, 90 participants completed the ESS and at 7 years, 45 completed it. EDS prevalence was 53% and 44%, respectively. No significant predictors in change in ESS score were found.

In another longitudinal, population-based study of EDS in a more advanced PD cohort, 232 patients with parkinsonism were assessed for EDS using a sleep questionnaire and ESS was later added to the study protocol (Gjerstad et al., 2006). Follow-up assessment occurred for 138 at 4 years, and 89 at 8 years. At baseline, 5.6% of the cohort had EDS, increasing to 22.5% at year 4% and 40.8% at year 8. The 8-year prevalence rate was 54.2%. Predictors of EDS included age, gender, and use of dopamine agonists. However, EDS did develop in patients without exposure to dopamine agonist, and in those cases EDS was related to motor disease severity (as measured by Hoehn and Yahr stage) (Gjerstad et al., 2006).

Studies examining the prevalence of EDS based on objective measurements are limited by their small sample size. What studies using MSLT are available indicate that in the general PD population without subjective daytime sleepiness, objective EDS may not be more likely in PD compared to controls, with mean sleep latencies of about 10–12 minutes in both groups and without significant differences. MSLT studies have found EDS in 13%–47% of patients without subjective complaints of EDS (Ataide et al., 2014). As for studies of PD patients with subjective sleepiness, there are few studies comparing MSLT findings in those patients to non-PD controls. In one study of PD patients with subjective EDS, up to 67% had objective evidence of EDS as well (Ataide et al., 2014). Sleep-onset REM periods on MSLT may be more predictive of subjective daytime EDS (Rye, Bliwise, Dihenia, & Gurecki, 2000), and there is certainly a subset of PD patients with narcolepsy-like hypersomnolence documented on MSLT.

Another proxy of daytime sleepiness is actigraphy, which measures movement. Actigraphy can be an accurate proxy of sleep, but also may reflect reduced mobility due to sleepiness (Kotschet et al., 2014). In a study of 85 PD patients and 21 age-matched non-PD controls studied, PD patients had significantly greater time spent napping compared to controls (Bolitho et al., 2013). Extent of daytime napping did not correlate with subjective EDS as assessed with the ESS.

Indeed, although in some studies a relationship between objective and subjective sleep measures has been demonstrated (Ataide et al., 2014; Monaca et al., 2006; Poryazova et al., 2010), other studies indicate a lack of consistent relationship between objective and subjective measures of EDS in PD (Bliwise et al., 2013; Bolitho et al., 2013; Chung et al., 2013; Compta et al., 2009). This may in part relate to a lack of sensitivity of objective measures or could reflect other PD symptoms that patients perceive as sleepiness (such as fatigue).

Etiology and differential diagnosis

There are several potential etiologies of daytime sleepiness in PD (Table 12.1; Fig. 12.1).

It may be a manifestation of underlying neurodegeneration involving wake-promoting regions in the brain. It may result in part from nighttime sleep problems, and in part from PD medications. Several neuropsychiatric symptoms are comorbid with EDS in PD that may reflect more severe underlying neurodegeneration, but could also be directly contributing to EDS as well. For example, hypersomnolence is a core feature of depression in some cases.

PD medications and EDS

Although a few studies have not demonstrated increased risk of EDS with dopamine agonist use (Ferreira, Prabhakar, & Kharbanda, 2014; Hu et al., 2011; Setthawatcharawanich et al., 2011; Stefansdottir, Gjerstad, Tysnes, & Larsen, 2012), including on objective testing (Ataide et al., 2014), there are nevertheless ample data to indicate that dopamine agonists are associated with increased risk of EDS (Oved et al., 2006; Poryazova et al., 2010; Valko et al., 2010).

Table 12.1 Potential contributors to EDS in PD.

Category	Contributor	Comment
Medications	Dopamine agonists	Although all dopamine agonists can cause hypersomnolence, data supporting this are stronger for pramipexole > rotigotine > ropinirole.
	Levodopa	Levodopa monotherapy is associated with EDS especially in more advanced PD, and can be exacerbated by concomitant therapy with dopamine agonists
	Entacapone	Entacapone likely contributes to EDS indirectly be increasing levodopa levels
	Non-PD meds	Sedating antidepressants, benzodiazepines
Nighttime sleep problems	Obstructive sleep apnea	See Chapter 8
	Insomnia	See Chapters 1 and 2
Neuropsychiatric symptoms	Depression, psychosis, cognitive dysfunction	Whether these are causative or comorbid to EDS in PD is not clear. Depression can manifest with EDS, and nocturnal psychosis could lead to EDS indirectly by disrupting nighttime sleep.
Underlying neurodegeneration	Brainstem/ diencephalic neurodegeneration	Degeneration of wake-promoting regions may cause or contribute to EDS in PD

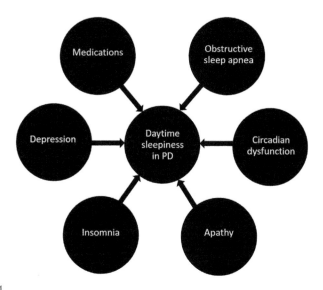

FIGURE 12.1

Contributors to excessive daytime sleepiness in PD.

In randomized trials, pramipexole (Goldman et al., 2013; Prudon et al., 2014) and rotigotine (Jankovic, Watts, Martin, & Boroojerdi, 2007; Watts et al., 2007) were both significantly more likely to cause hypersomnolence compared to placebo. Pramipexole was more likely to cause hypersomnolence compared to other PD drugs including rasagiline (Viallet, Pitel, Lancrenon, & Blin, 2013) and levodopa (Parkinson Study Group CALM Cohort Investigators, 2009). Indeed, the rate of hypersomnolence was almost twice as high in pramipexole-treated patients compared to levodopa (Parkinson Study Group CALM Cohort Investigators, 2009). Pramipexole is renally cleared, and a risk factor of pramipexole-induced hypersomnolence is thus renal dysfunction (Baba et al., 2011). The incidence of EDS in open-label studies of PD patients treated with rotigotine was 23%–30% per patient-year (Elmer, Surmann, Boroojerdi, & Jankovic, 2012; LeWitt et al., 2013). In randomized, placebo-controlled studies, ropinirole did not show significantly higher rates of hypersomnolence compared to placebo (Pahwa et al., 2007; Ray Chaudhuri et al., 2012; Rektorova et al., 2008) but other data as well as anecdotal evidence in clinical practice indicate that hypersomnolence is a risk in ropinirole-treated patients. Extended-release formulations may be associated with less EDS than immediate-release formulations but data are limited (Dusek et al., 2010).

As for other PD drugs, rasagiline is not associated with increased risk of EDS compared to placebo (Hauser et al., 2014). Entacapone may also increase risk of EDS but, again, data are limited (Koller, Guarnieri, Hubble, Rabinowicz, & Silver, 2005). Cumulatively, PD dopaminergic exposure in aggregate increases risk of EDS; levodopa equivalent daily dose predicts subjective sleepiness (Chung et al., 2013). As for PD drugs that could actually improve EDS, an open-label study indicated that selegiline improves EDS (Lyons et al., 2010), possibly through methamphetamine properties of its metabolites. Amantadine is also less likely to cause EDS than the dopaminergic drugs; indeed, it has been suggested as a potential treatment for fatigue in other populations, but data supporting its utility in this regard are insufficient (Taus, Giuliani, Pucci, D'Amico, & Solari, 2003).

Nocturnal sleep problems and EDS

In many patients, EDS is not substantially explained by nighttime sleep problems (Goldman et al., 2013). Indeed, many studies have not shown a clear relationship between subjective or objective nighttime sleep and daytime sleepiness. In a study that examined objective measures of daytime sleepiness using multiple sleep latency test, mean sleep latency was not related to subjective sleepiness but rather most strongly predicted by disease duration and motor severity (Wienecke et al., 2012).

Having said that, poor nighttime sleep likely contributes to EDS at least in some patients (Ataide et al., 2014), and certain sleep disorders are more common in PD patients with EDS versus those without. PD patients with Rapid eye movement sleep behavior disorder (RBD) are more likely to have EDS compared to those without (Poryazova, Oberholzer, Baumann, & Bassetti, 2013; Rolinski et al., 2014). In one study, PD patients with RBD had shorter MSL, though neither had an MSL in the abnormal range (Plomhause et al., 2013). RLS may be another sleep disorder that is associated with EDS in PD. Although one study showed no relationship between RLS and EDS (Bhalsing, Suresh, Muthane, & Pal, 2013), another reported RLS to be an independent predictor of EDS (Moreno-Lopez et al., 2011), and in another study RLS severity correlated with EDS (Verbaan, van Rooden, van Hilten, & Rijsman, 2010). Circadian abnormalities are also seen in PD patients with EDS; one study showed a lower amplitude of melatonin rhythm (Videnovic et al., 2014). See Chapter 9 for more on circadian abnormalities in PD and how they may contribute to EDS. Another sleep disorder that may contribute to EDS in PD is sleep apnea. Although some studies have not shown a relationship between AHI and either objective or subjective measures of EDS in PD (Cochen De Cock et al., 2010, 2014; Lelieveld et al., 2012; Nomura, Inoue, Kobayashi, Namba, & Nakashima, 2013; Suzuki et al., 2008; Trotti & Bliwise, 2010; Valko et al., 2010), other studies have indicated that at least in some patients, apnea-hypopnea index (AHI) predicts subjective sleepiness (Norlinah et al., 2009; Poryazova et al., 2010; Shpirer et al., 2006). Continuous positive airway pressure should certainly be initiated in PD patients with OSA and EDS (see Chapter 8 for more information on sleep disordered breathing in PD).

Comorbid nonmotor manifestations, underlying neurodegeneration, and EDS

Several nonmotor manifestations are more common in PD patients with EDS versus those without, including neuropsychiatric and autonomic symptoms. For example,

EDS is more common in PD patients with cognitive dysfunction and dementia (Archibald, Clarke, Mosimann, & Burn, 2011; Boddy et al., 2007; Compta et al., 2009; Goldman et al., 2013; Larsson et al., 2010). Similarly, EDS is more common in PD patients with depression (Margis et al., 2009), and EDS predicts depression in PD (Suzuki et al., 2008, 2009).

As discussed in Chapter 4 on nocturnal psychosis in PD, psychosis is a strong predictor of EDS (Barnes, Connelly, Wiggs, Boubert, & Maravic, 2010), and PD psychosis is more common in PD patients with EDS compared to those without (Lee & Weintraub, 2012; Verbaan et al., 2009). Longitudinally, EDS predicts onset of psychosis (Zhu, van Hilten, Putter, & Marinus, 2013) though this is likely multi-factorial (Gallagher et al., 2011; Lee & Weintraub, 2012; Pacchetti et al., 2005) and to what degree it is causative, versus reflecting more severe neurodegeneration, is not clear. Similarly, PD patients with EDS are more likely to have autonomic dysfunction (Jain et al., 2011; Kurtis, Rodriguez-Blazquez, Martinez-Martin, & ELEP Group, 2013; Verbaan et al., 2007).

PD patients with EDS are also more likely to have psychiatric symptoms as well (Verbaan et al., 2008). In a study attempting to examine the relationship between depression, anxiety, and EDS, 120 PD patients were assessed with the Pittsburgh Sleep Quality Index (PSQI) the ESS. The strongest predictors of EDS were male sex, disease duration, and comorbid anxiety (Borek et al., 2006).

As mentioned, whether all these comorbidities are causative of EDS or rather if they are both just markers of more severe underlying neurodegeneration requires further investigation. It is possible that both of these relationships may be true to some extent. Data to support the idea that EDS is at least to some extent a reflection of more severe neurodegeneration in PD come from structural imaging studies. In volumetric MRI studies comparing PD patients with EDS compared to those without, PD patients with EDS had lower volumes in several regions including the frontal, temporal, occipital lobes, nucleus basalis of Meynert (Kato et al., 2012) and middle cerebellar peduncle (Gama et al., 2010). PD patients with EDS also were shown to have reduced fractional anisotropy in the fornix on diffusion tensor imaging (Matsui et al., 2006).

Hypocretin neurons degenerate in narcolepsy, a disorder characterized by profound hypersomnia. The narcolepsy-like hypersomnolence seen in some PD patients has prompted evaluation of hypocretin neuronal integrity in PD. In a small study of 11 PD patients compared to five non-PD controls, significantly greater loss of hypocretin neurons was seen in the PD group, and the degree of loss correlated with disease severity (Thannickal, Lai, & Siegel, 2007). CSF hypocretin levels have also been examined in PD. One study did not find a relationship between EDS and CSF hypocretin (Compta et al., 2009). In another study that examined hypocretin levels in CSF in 31 PD patients compared to 13 non-PD controls, no difference between the PD and control group was found in CSF hypocretin levels, or between advanced and early PD. However, CSF hypocretin levels did correlate with mean sleep latency in the PD group (Wienecke et al., 2012).

Consequences and complications

EDS in PD is associated with worse QOL (Gallagher, Lees, & Schrag, 2010; Havlikova et al., 2011; Sobreira-Neto et al., 2017), and independently predicts worse health-related quality of life (QOL) (Visser et al., 2008). As discussed earlier, EDS is associated with several other nonmotor manifestations. Not only are cognitive decline and psychosis more common in PD patients with EDS compared to those without, but also EDS predicts emergence of these other nonmotor manifestations. PD patients with EDS are at higher risk of cognitive decline (Goldman, Stebbins, Leung, TilleyB, & Goetz, 2014) and dementia on follow-up (Zhu, van Hilten, & Marinus, 2014). EDS also predicts onset of psychosis (Zhu et al., 2013). However, cognitive dysfunction and psychosis are both likely multifactorial (Gallagher et al., 2011; Lee & Weintraub, 2012; Pacchetti et al., 2005) and to what degree EDS is causative, contributes, and/or is just a marker of more severe neurodegeneration that in turn manifests with psychosis and cognitive impairment, is not clear.

There are safety concerns related to EDS in PD. PD patients with daytime sleepiness demonstrate impaired driving performance in the context of auditory-verbal distractors (Uc et al., 2006). PD patients with EDS have higher risk of motor vehicle accidents. 8% of PD patients of 5210 with a driver's license reported episodes of sudden onset of sleep and almost one-third had accidents or near-accidents related to sleepiness (Meindorfner et al., 2005). Importantly, subjective sleepiness does not accurately predict sudden onset sleep (Ferreira et al., 2006). The lack of insight into sleepiness in PD also reflects in less safe decisions during driving (Crizzle, Myers, Roy, & Almeida, 2013). As mentioned, EDS in PD can be caused by dopamine agonists and indeed, dopamine agonists are a risk factor for sudden onset sleep episodes in PD that are not always predictable (Avorn et al., 2005) and may thus be a risk factor for motor vehicle accidents in PD.

Another adverse consequence of EDS is that it is associated with increased caregiver burden in PD as well (Ozdilek. & Gunal. , 2012).

Management

Several treatment strategies may be considered for PD patients with EDS (Table 12.2).

The Movement Disorders Society has issued a taskforce-synthesized evidence-based review of nonmotor symptoms in PD (Seppi et al., 2019). The taskforce did not find sufficient evidence to definitively recommend pharmacologic therapy for EDS in PD. However, they indicated that the wake-promoting agent modafinil was possibly useful. Indeed, a meta-analysis of three randomized placebo-controlled trials did find significant improvements in EDS, as assessed with ESS, in PD.

As for methylphenidate, it has mainly been studied with changes in fatigue (not EDS) as the outcome. It could be considered in some PD patients with EDS, though risk of cardiovascular side effects should be carefully weighed (Seppi et al., 2011).

Table 12.2 Management of EDS in PD.

Category	Drug	Comment
Wake-promoting agents	Modafinil	Small randomized trials have supported benefit of modafinil in some patients with EDS. Data supporting utility of other agents are markedly limited.
	Methamphetamine	
	Caffeine	
	Selegiline	Morning dosing of selegiline can improve sleepiness in PD while also improving motor function
Treatment of nocturnal sleep	CPAP	CPAP should be encouraged in PD patients with OSA as treatment could improve EDS
	Sodium oxybate	Sodium oxybate may improve nighttime sleep but data on its use in PD are limited, and with very limited safety data for it in PD, its use should be weighed carefully.
	Sedative hypnotics	In patients with sleep onset and maintenance insomnia, improving nighttime sleep could reduce EDS. On the other hand, residual sleepiness resulting from these drugs is a risk that must be monitored for closely with initiation of any such drugs.
Behavioral/environmental	Exercise	Preliminary data indicate exercise may improve EDS in PD
	Bright light therapy	Preliminary data indicate therapeutic bright light therapy may improve EDS in PD

The taskforce also indicated that caffeine is considered "investigational" for treatment of EDS in PD. One randomized, placebo-controlled trial of caffeine in PD showed nonsignificant improvements in EDS, as assessed with ESS (Postuma et al., 2017). Of note, the task force also indicated that continuous positive airway pressure (CPAP) was likely efficacious for treatment of EDS in PD patients with OSA (Seppi et al., 2019). See Chapter 8 for more information on sleep-disordered breathing in PD. Sodium oxybate is a medication used to treat narcolepsy; it increases stage 3 sleep (see Chapter 13) and is thought to possibly improve EDS via its effects on nighttime sleep. A small pilot randomized placebo-controlled cross-over trial (2–4 week washout period) of sodium oxybate in 12 PD patients used MSLT as the primary outcome measure (Buchele et al., 2018). Mean sleep latency increased by 2.9 minutes, which was statistically significant but of unclear clinical significance. ESS did significantly decrease as well.

Treatment of comorbidities often seen in EDS may improve EDS as well. For example, a post hoc analysis of pooled data from two randomized, double-blind controlled studies of pimavanserin for PD psychosis (Cummings et al., 2013) included data from 187 PD patients who received pimavanserin and 187 who received placebo (Patel et al., 2018). Improvement in EDS, as measured by the daytime symptom subscore of the Scales for Outcomes in Parkinson's-SLEEP (SCOPA-SLEEP) was observed in one of the trials and there was a trend toward significant improvement among patients who had reported both impaired nighttime sleep and daytime sleepiness. Similarly, treatment of comorbidities such as depression could anecdotally improve daytime energy in some patients as well. Atomoxetine, a selective norepinephrine reuptake inhibitor, may improve EDS as well, though data are limited (Weintraub et al., 2010). Finally, in some patients, strategic napping in the late morning or early afternoon, for brief periods (20 minutes or less), could help EDS. However, caution must be taken to time naps and limit duration to minimize risk of inducing insomnia or otherwise affecting nighttime sleep.

As for PD drugs that could actually improve EDS, an open-label study indicated selegiline improves EDS (Lyons et al., 2010), possibly through methamphetamine properties of its metabolites.

Although data are limited, preliminary reports indicate that bright light therapy may be a useful treatment for EDS in PD. A small randomized trial of bright light (10,000 lux) therapy versus dim light therapy administered twice a day for 2 weeks was conducted in 31 PD patients (Videnovic et al., 2017). The bright light therapy arm demonstrated improved EDS as assessed by ESS, as well as improvement in nighttime sleep as assessed with the PSQI. Exercise is another area of investigation as a potential means of improving EDS in PD (Cusso, Donald, & Khoo, 2016).

Illustrative case in context

The case presented is a 67-year-old man with a clinical history consistent with EDS. This is affecting his quality of life and putting him at increased risk for motor vehicle accidents. The history indicates mild apathy as well, but no depression. There is a history of occasional snoring and given that he has unrefreshing sleep, a polysomnogram is indicated to rule out obstructive sleep apnea. Pramipexole should be tapered and stopped as it can cause hypersomnolence. Although there are limited data supporting the utility of exercise in treating EDS in PD, some physical activity would be useful as part of his general PD treatment regimen and could possibly improve his EDS as well. Bright light therapy is another possible consideration for him.

References

Abbott, R. D., Ross, G. W., White, L. R., Tanner, C. M., Masaki, K. H., Nelson, J. S., et al. (2005). Excessive daytime sleepiness and subsequent development of Parkinson disease. *Neurology, 65*(9), 1442–1446.

Adler, C. H., Hentz, J. G., Shill, H. A., Sabbagh, M. N., Driver-Dunckley, E., Evidente, V. G., et al. (2011). Probable RBD is increased in Parkinson's disease but not in essential tremor or restless legs syndrome. *Parkinsonism & Related Disorders, 17*(6), 456–458.

Amara, A. W., Chahine, L. M., Caspell-Garcia, C., Long, J. D., Coffey, C., Hogl, B., et al. (2017). Longitudinal assessment of excessive daytime sleepiness in early Parkinson's disease. *Journal of Neurology, Neurosurgery & Psychiatry, 88*(8), 653–662.

American Academy of Sleep Medicine. (2014). *International classification of sleep disorders* (3rd ed.). Darien, IL: American Academy of Sleep Medicine.

Archibald, N. K., Clarke, M. P., Mosimann, U. P., & Burn, D. J. (2011). Visual symptoms in Parkinson's disease and Parkinson's disease dementia. *Movement Disorders: Official Journal of the Movement Disorder Society, 26*(13), 2387–2395.

Ataide, M., Franco, C. M., & Lins, O. G. (2014). Daytime sleepiness and Parkinson's disease: The contribution of the multiple sleep latency test. *Sleep Disorders, 2014*, 767181.

Avorn, J., Schneeweiss, S., Sudarsky, L. R., Benner, J., Kiyota, Y., Levin, R., et al. (2005). Sudden uncontrollable somnolence and medication use in Parkinson disease. *Archives of Neurology, 62*(8), 1242–1248.

Baba, Y., Higuchi, M. A., Fukuyama, K., Abe, H., Uehara, Y., Inoue, T., et al. (2011). Effect of chronic kidney disease on excessive daytime sleepiness in Parkinson disease. *European Journal of Neurology: The Official Journal of the European Federation of Neurological Societies, 18*(11), 1299–1303.

Barnes, J., Connelly, V., Wiggs, L., Boubert, L., & Maravic, K. (2010). Sleep patterns in Parkinson's disease patients with visual hallucinations. *The International Journal of Neuroscience, 120*(8), 564–569.

Bhalsing, K., Suresh, K., Muthane, U. B., & Pal, P. K. (2013). Prevalence and profile of restless legs syndrome in Parkinson's disease and other neurodegenerative disorders: A case-control study. *Parkinsonism & Related Disorders, 19*(4), 426–430.

Bjornara, K. A., Dietrichs, E., & Toft, M. (2014). Clinical features associated with sleep disturbances in Parkinson's disease. *Clinical Neurology and Neurosurgery, 124*, 37–43.

Bliwise, D. L., Trotti, L. M., Juncos, J. J., Factor, S. A., Freeman, A., & Rye, D. B. (2013). Daytime REM sleep in Parkinson's disease. *Parkinsonism & Related Disorders, 19*(1), 101–103.

Boddy, F., Rowan, E. N., Lett, D., O'Brien, J. T., McKeith, I. G., & Burn, D. J. (2007). Subjectively reported sleep quality and excessive daytime somnolence in Parkinson's disease with and without dementia, dementia with Lewy bodies and Alzheimer's disease. *International Journal of Geriatric Psychiatry, 22*(6), 529–535.

Bolitho, S. J., Naismith, S. L., Salahuddin, P., Terpening, Z., Grunstein, R. R., & Lewis, S. J. (2013). Objective measurement of daytime napping, cognitive dysfunction and subjective sleepiness in Parkinson's disease. *PLoS One, 8*(11), e81233.

Borek, L. L., Kohn, R., & Friedman, J. H. (2006). Mood and sleep in Parkinson's disease. *The Journal of Clinical Psychiatry, 67*(6), 958–963.

Breen, D. P., Williams-Gray, C. H., Mason, S. L., Foltynie, T., & Barker, R. A. (2013). Excessive daytime sleepiness and its risk factors in incident Parkinson's disease. *Journal of Neurology, Neurosurgery & Psychiatry, 84*(2), 233–234.

Buchele, F., Hackius, M., Schreglmann, S. R., Omlor, W., Werth, E., Maric, A., et al. (2018). Sodium oxybate for excessive daytime sleepiness and sleep disturbance in Parkinson disease: A randomized clinical trial. *JAMA Neurology, 75*(1), 114–118.

Chotinaiwattarakul, W., Dayalu, P., Chervin, R. D., & Albin, R. L. (2011). Risk of sleep-disordered breathing in Parkinson's disease. *Sleep & Breathing = Schlaf & Atmung, 15*(3), 471–478.

Chung, S., Bohnen, N. I., Albin, R. L., Frey, K. A., Muller, M. L., & Chervin, R. D. (2013). Insomnia and sleepiness in Parkinson disease: Associations with symptoms and comorbidities. *Journal of Clinical Sleep Medicine: Official Publication of the American Academy of Sleep Medicine, 9*(11), 1131–1137.

Cochen De Cock, V., Abouda, M., Leu, S., Oudiette, D., Roze, E., Vidailhet, M., et al. (2010). Is obstructive sleep apnea a problem in Parkinson's disease? *Sleep Medicine, 11*(3), 247–252.

Cochen De Cock, V., Bayard, S., Jaussent, I., Charif, M., Grini, M., Langenier, M. C., et al. (2014). Daytime sleepiness in Parkinson's disease: A reappraisal. *PLoS One, 9*(9), e107278.

Compta, Y., Santamaria, J., Ratti, L., Tolosa, E., Iranzo, A., Munoz, E., et al. (2009). Cerebrospinal hypocretin, daytime sleepiness and sleep architecture in Parkinson's disease dementia. *Brain: Journal of Neurology, 132*(Pt 12), 3308–3317.

Crizzle, A. M., Myers, A. M., Roy, E. A., & Almeida, Q. J. (2013). Drivers with Parkinson's disease: Are the symptoms of PD associated with restricted driving practices? *Journal of Neurology, 260*(10), 2562–2568.

Cummings, J., Isaacson, S., Mills, R., Williams, H., Chi-Burris, K., Corbett, A., et al. (2013). Pimavanserin for patients with Parkinson's disease psychosis: A randomised, placebo-controlled phase 3 trial. *Lancet*.

Cusso, M. E., Donald, K. J., & Khoo, T. K. (2016). The impact of physical activity on non-motor symptoms in Parkinson's disease: A systematic review. *Frontiers of Medicine, 3*, 35.

Dhawan, V., Dhoat, S., Williams, A. J., Dimarco, A., Pal, S., Forbes, A., et al. (2006). The range and nature of sleep dysfunction in untreated Parkinson's disease (PD). A comparative controlled clinical study using the Parkinson's disease sleep scale and selective polysomnography. *Journal of the Neurological Sciences, 248*(1–2), 158–162.

Dusek, P., Buskova, J., Ruzicka, E., Majerova, V., Srp, A., Jech, R., et al. (2010). Effects of ropinirole prolonged-release on sleep disturbances and daytime sleepiness in Parkinson disease. *Clinical Neuropharmacology, 33*(4), 186–190.

Elmer, L. W., Surmann, E., Boroojerdi, B., & Jankovic, J. (2012). Long-term safety and tolerability of rotigotine transdermal system in patients with early-stage idiopathic Parkinson's disease: A prospective, open-label extension study. *Parkinsonism & Related Disorders, 18*(5), 488–493.

Ferreira, J. J., Desboeuf, K., Galitzky, M., Thalamas, C., Brefel-Courbon, C., Fabre, N., et al. (2006). Sleep disruption, daytime somnolence and 'sleep attacks' in Parkinson's disease: A clinical survey in PD patients and age-matched healthy volunteers. *European Journal of Neurology: The Official Journal of the European Federation of Neurological Societies, 13*(3), 209–214.

Ferreira, T., Prabhakar, S., & Kharbanda, P. S. (2014). Sleep disturbances in drug naive Parkinson's disease (PD) patients and effect of levodopa on sleep. *Annals of Indian Academy of Neurology, 17*(4), 416–419.

Gallagher, D. A., Lees, A. J., & Schrag, A. (2010). What are the most important nonmotor symptoms in patients with Parkinson's disease and are we missing them? *Movement Disorders: Official Journal of the Movement Disorder Society, 25*(15), 2493–2500.

Gallagher, D. A., Parkkinen, L., O'Sullivan, S. S., Spratt, A., Shah, A., Davey, C. C., et al. (2011). Testing an aetiological model of visual hallucinations in Parkinson's disease. *Brain: Journal of Neurology, 134*(Pt 11), 3299–3309.

Gama, R. L., Tavora, D. G., Bomfim, R. C., Silva, C. E., de Bruin, V. M., & de Bruin, P. F. (2010). Sleep disturbances and brain MRI morphometry in Parkinson's disease, multiple system atrophy and progressive supranuclear palsy - a comparative study. *Parkinsonism & Related Disorders, 16*(4), 275−279.

Gerbin, M., Viner, A. S., & Louis, E. D. (2012). Sleep in essential tremor: A comparison with normal controls and Parkinson's disease patients. *Parkinsonism & Related Disorders, 18*(3), 279−284.

Ghorayeb, I., Loundou, A., Auquier, P., Dauvilliers, Y., Bioulac, B., & Tison, F. (2007). A nationwide survey of excessive daytime sleepiness in Parkinson's disease in France. *Movement Disorders: Official Journal of the Movement Disorder Society, 22*(11), 1567−1572.

Gjerstad, M. D., Alves, G., Wentzel-Larsen, T., Aarsland, D., & Larsen, J. P. (2006). Excessive daytime sleepiness in Parkinson disease: Is it the drugs or the disease? *Neurology, 67*(5), 853−858.

Goetz, C. G., Tilley, B. C., Shaftman, S. R., Stebbins, G. T., Fahn, S., Martinez-Martin, P., et al. (2008). Movement disorder society-sponsored revision of the unified Parkinson's disease rating scale (MDS-UPDRS): Scale presentation and clinimetric testing results. *Movement Disorders: Official Journal of the Movement Disorder Society, 23*(15), 2129−2170.

Goldman, J. G., Ghode, R. A., Ouyang, B., Bernard, B., Goetz, C. G., & Stebbins, G. T. (2013). Dissociations among daytime sleepiness, nighttime sleep, and cognitive status in Parkinson's disease. *Parkinsonism & Related Disorders, 19*(9), 806−811.

Goldman, J. G., Stebbins, G. T., Leung, V., Tilley, B. C., & Goetz, C. G. (2014). Relationships among cognitive impairment, sleep, and fatigue in Parkinson's disease using the MDS-UPDRS. *Parkinsonism & Related Disorders.*

Goulart, F. O., Godke, B. A., Borges, V., Azevedo-Silva, S. M., Mendes, M. F., Cendoroglo, M. S., et al. (2009). Fatigue in a cohort of geriatric patients with and without Parkinson's disease. *Brazilian Journal of Medical and Biological Research = Revista Brasileira De Pesquisas Medicas e Biologicas/Sociedade Brasileira De Biofisica, 42*(8), 771−775.

Hagell, P., & Broman, J. E. (2007). Measurement properties and hierarchical item structure of the Epworth Sleepiness Scale in Parkinson's disease. *Journal of Sleep Research, 16*(1), 102−109.

Happe, S., Baier, P. C., Bachmann, C. G., Helmschmied, M. D., & Paulus, W. (2008). Nocturnal restlessness and distressing dreams in patients with early Parkinson's disease: Role of the Parkinson's disease sleep scale (PDSS). *Somnologie, 12*(1), 50−55.

Hauser, R. A., Silver, D., Choudhry, A., Eyal, E., Isaacson, S., & ANDANTE study investigators. (2014). Randomized, controlled trial of rasagiline as an add-on to dopamine agonists in Parkinson's disease. *Movement Disorders: Official Journal of the Movement Disorder Society, 29*(8), 1028−1034.

Havlikova, E., van Dijk, J. P., Nagyova, I., Rosenberger, J., Middel, B., Dubayova, T., et al. (2011). The impact of sleep and mood disorders on quality of life in Parkinson's disease patients. *Journal of Neurology, 258*(12), 2222−2229.

Hu, M., Cooper, J., Beamish, R., Jones, E., Butterworth, R., Catterall, L., et al. (2011). How well do we recognise non-motor symptoms in a British Parkinson's disease population? *Journal of Neurology, 258*(8), 1513−1517.

Jain, S., Siegle, G. J., Gu, C., Moore, C. G., Ivanco, L. S., Studenski, S., et al. (2011). Pupillary unrest correlates with arousal symptoms and motor signs in Parkinson disease. *Movement Disorders: Official Journal of the Movement Disorder Society, 26*(7), 1344−1347.

Jankovic, J., Watts, R. L., Martin, W., & Boroojerdi, B. (2007). Transdermal rotigotine: Double-blind, placebo-controlled trial in Parkinson disease. *Archives of Neurology, 64*(5), 676–682.

Johns, M. W. (1991). A new method for measuring daytime sleepiness: The Epworth sleepiness scale. *Sleep, 14*(6), 540–545.

Jongwanasiri, S., Prayoonwiwat, N., Pisarnpong, A., Srivanitchapoom, P., & Chotinaiwattarakul, W. (2014). Evaluation of sleep disorders in Parkinson's disease: A comparison between physician diagnosis and self-administered questionnaires. *Journal of the Medical Association of Thailand = Chotmaihet Thangphaet, 97*(Suppl. 3), S68–S77.

Kato, S., Watanabe, H., Senda, J., Hirayama, M., Ito, M., Atsuta, N., et al. (2012). Widespread cortical and subcortical brain atrophy in Parkinson's disease with excessive daytime sleepiness. *Journal of Neurology, 259*(2), 318–326.

Knipe, M. D., Wickremaratchi, M. M., Wyatt-Haines, E., Morris, H. R., & Ben-Shlomo, Y. (2011). Quality of life in young- compared with late-onset Parkinson's disease. *Movement Disorders: Official Journal of the Movement Disorder Society, 26*(11), 2011–2018.

Koller, W., Guarnieri, M., Hubble, J., Rabinowicz, A. L., & Silver, D. (2005). An open-label evaluation of the tolerability and safety of Stalevo (carbidopa, levodopa and entacapone) in Parkinson's disease patients experiencing wearing-off. *Journal of Neural Transmission, 112*(2), 221–230.

Kotschet, K., Johnson, W., McGregor, S., Kettlewell, J., Kyoong, A., O'Driscoll, D. M., et al. (2014). Daytime sleep in Parkinson's disease measured by episodes of immobility. *Parkinsonism & Related Disorders, 20*(6), 578–583.

Kurtis, M. M., Rodriguez-Blazquez, C., Martinez-Martin, P., & ELEP Group. (2013). Relationship between sleep disorders and other non-motor symptoms in Parkinson's disease. *Parkinsonism & Related Disorders, 19*(12), 1152–1155.

Larsson, V., Aarsland, D., Ballard, C., Minthon, L., & Londos, E. (2010). The effect of memantine on sleep behaviour in dementia with Lewy bodies and Parkinson's disease dementia. *International Journal of Geriatric Psychiatry, 25*(10), 1030–1038.

Lee, A. H., & Weintraub, D. (2012). Psychosis in Parkinson's disease without dementia: Common and comorbid with other non-motor symptoms. *Movement Disorders: Official Journal of the Movement Disorder Society, 27*(7), 858–863.

Lelieveld, I. M., Muller, M. L., Bohnen, N. I., Koeppe, R. A., Chervin, R. D., Frey, K. A., et al. (2012). The role of serotonin in sleep disordered breathing associated with Parkinson disease: A correlative [11C]DASB PET imaging study. *PLoS One, 7*(7), e40166.

LeWitt, P. A., Boroojerdi, B., Surmann, E., Poewe, W., & SP716 Study Group, & SP715 Study Group. (2013). Rotigotine transdermal system for long-term treatment of patients with advanced Parkinson's disease: Results of two open-label extension studies, CLEOPATRA-PD and PREFER. *Journal of Neural Transmission, 120*(7), 1069–1081.

Littner, M. R., Kushida, C., Wise, M., Davila, D. G., Morgenthaler, T., Lee-Chiong, T., et al. (2005). Practice parameters for clinical use of the multiple sleep latency test and the maintenance of wakefulness test. *Sleep, 28*(1), 113–121.

Louter, M., van der Marck, M. A., Pevernagie, D. A., Munneke, M., Bloem, B. R., & Overeem, S. (2013). Sleep matters in Parkinson's disease: Use of a priority list to assess the presence of sleep disturbances. *European Journal of Neurology: The Official Journal of the European Federation of Neurological Societies, 20*(2), 259–265.

Lyons, K. E., Friedman, J. H., Hermanowicz, N., Isaacson, S. H., Hauser, R. A., Hersh, B. P., et al. (2010). Orally disintegrating selegiline in Parkinson patients with dopamine agonist-related adverse effects. *Clinical Neuropharmacology, 33*(1), 5–10.

Margis, R., Donis, K., Schonwald, S. V., Fagondes, S. C., Monte, T., Martin-Martinez, P., et al. (2009). Psychometric properties of the Parkinson's disease sleep scale–Brazilian version. *Parkinsonism & Related Disorders, 15*(7), 495–499.

Marinus, J., Visser, M., van Hilten, J. J., Lammers, G. J., & Stiggelbout, A. M. (2003). Assessment of sleep and sleepiness in Parkinson disease. *Sleep, 26*(8), 1049–1054.

Matsui, H., Nishinaka, K., Oda, M., Niikawa, H., Komatsu, K., Kubori, T., et al. (2006). Disruptions of the fornix fiber in Parkinsonian patients with excessive daytime sleepiness. *Parkinsonism & Related Disorders, 12*(5), 319–322.

Meindorfner, C., Korner, Y., Moller, J. C., Stiasny-Kolster, K., Oertel, W. H., & Kruger, H. P. (2005). Driving in Parkinson's disease: Mobility, accidents, and sudden onset of sleep at the wheel. *Movement Disorders: Official Journal of the Movement Disorder Society, 20*(7), 832–842.

Monaca, C., Duhamel, A., Jacquesson, J. M., Ozsancak, C., Destee, A., Guieu, J. D., et al. (2006). Vigilance troubles in Parkinson's disease: A subjective and objective polysomnographic study. *Sleep Medicine, 7*(5), 448–453.

Moreno-Lopez, C., Santamaria, J., Salamero, M., Del Sorbo, F., Albanese, A., Pellecchia, M. T., et al. (2011). Excessive daytime sleepiness in multiple system atrophy (SLEEMSA study). *Archives of Neurology, 68*(2), 223–230.

Nomura, T., Inoue, Y., Kobayashi, M., Namba, K., & Nakashima, K. (2013). Characteristics of obstructive sleep apnea in patients with Parkinson's disease. *Journal of the Neurological Sciences, 327*(1–2), 22–24.

Norlinah, M. I., Afidah, K. N., Noradina, A. T., Shamsul, A. S., Hamidon, B. B., Sahathevan, R., et al. (2009). Sleep disturbances in Malaysian patients with Parkinson's disease using polysomnography and PDSS. *Parkinsonism & Related Disorders, 15*(9), 670–674.

Oved, D., Ziv, I., Treves, T. A., Paleacu, D., Melamed, E., & Djaldetti, R. (2006). Effect of dopamine agonists on fatigue and somnolence in Parkinson's disease. *Movement Disorders: Official Journal of the Movement Disorder Society, 21*(8), 1257–1261.

Ozdilek, B., & Gunal, D. I. (2012). Motor and non-motor symptoms in Turkish patients with Parkinson's disease affecting family caregiver burden and quality of life. *The Journal of Neuropsychiatry and Clinical Neurosciences, 24*(4), 478–483.

Pacchetti, C., Manni, R., Zangaglia, R., Mancini, F., Marchioni, E., Tassorelli, C., et al. (2005). Relationship between hallucinations, delusions, and rapid eye movement sleep behavior disorder in Parkinson's disease. *Movement Disorders: Official Journal of the Movement Disorder Society, 20*(11), 1439–1448.

Pahwa, R., Stacy, M. A., Factor, S. A., Lyons, K. E., Stocchi, F., Hersh, B. P., et al. (2007). Ropinirole 24-hour prolonged release: Randomized, controlled study in advanced Parkinson disease. *Neurology, 68*(14), 1108–1115.

Parkinson Study Group CALM Cohort Investigators. (2009). Long-term effect of initiating pramipexole vs levodopa in early Parkinson disease. *Archives of Neurology, 66*(5), 563–570.

Patel, N., LeWitt, P., Neikrug, A. B., Kesslak, P., Coate, B., & Ancoli-Israel, S. (2018). Nighttime sleep and daytime sleepiness improved with pimavanserin during treatment of Parkinson's disease psychosis. *Clinical Neuropharmacology, 41*(6), 210–215.

Plomhause, L., Dujardin, K., Duhamel, A., Delliaux, M., Derambure, P., Defebvre, L., et al. (2013). Rapid eye movement sleep behavior disorder in treatment-naive Parkinson disease patients. *Sleep Medicine.*

Poryazova, R., Benninger, D., Waldvogel, D., & Bassetti, C. L. (2010). Excessive daytime sleepiness in Parkinson's disease: Characteristics and determinants. *European Neurology, 63*(3), 129−135.

Poryazova, R., Oberholzer, M., Baumann, C. R., & Bassetti, C. L. (2013). REM sleep behavior disorder in Parkinson's disease: A questionnaire-based survey. *Journal of Clinical Sleep Medicine: Official Publication of the American Academy of Sleep Medicine, 9*(1), 55−59.

Postuma, R. B., Anang, J., Pelletier, A., Joseph, L., Moscovich, M., Grimes, D., et al. (2017). Caffeine as symptomatic treatment for Parkinson disease (Cafe-PD): A randomized trial. *Neurology, 89*(17), 1795−1803.

Prudon, B., Duncan, G. W., Khoo, T. K., Yarnall, A. J., & Anderson, K. N. (2014). Primary sleep disorder prevalence in patients with newly diagnosed Parkinson's disease. *Movement Disorders: Official Journal of the Movement Disorder Society, 29*(2), 259−262.

Ray Chaudhuri, K., Martinez-Martin, P., Rolfe, K. A., Cooper, J., Rockett, C. B., Giorgi, L., et al. (2012). Improvements in nocturnal symptoms with ropinirole prolonged release in patients with advanced Parkinson's disease. *European Journal of Neurology: The Official Journal of the European Federation of Neurological Societies, 19*(1), 105−113.

Rektorova, I., Balaz, M., Svatova, J., Zarubova, K., Honig, I., Dostal, V., et al. (2008). Effects of ropinirole on nonmotor symptoms of Parkinson disease: A prospective multicenter study. *Clinical Neuropharmacology, 31*(5), 261−266.

Rolinski, M., Szewczyk-Krolikowski, K., Tomlinson, P. R., Nithi, K., Talbot, K., Ben-Shlomo, Y., et al. (2014). REM sleep behaviour disorder is associated with worse quality of life and other non-motor features in early Parkinson's disease. *Journal of Neurology, Neurosurgery & Psychiatry, 85*(5), 560−566.

Rye, D. B., Bliwise, D. L., Dihenia, B., & Gurecki, P. (2000). FAST TRACK: Daytime sleepiness in Parkinson's disease. *Journal of Sleep Research, 9*(1), 63−69.

Seppi, K., Ray Chaudhuri, K., Coelho, M., Fox, S. H., Katzenschlager, R., Perez Lloret, S., et al. (2019). Update on treatments for nonmotor symptoms of Parkinson's disease-an evidence-based medicine review. *Movement Disorders: Official Journal of the Movement Disorder Society, 34*(2), 180−198.

Seppi, K., Weintraub, D., Coelho, M., Perez-Lloret, S., Fox, S. H., Katzenschlager, R., et al. (2011). The movement disorder society evidence-based medicine review update: Treatments for the non-motor symptoms of Parkinson's disease. *Movement Disorders: Official Journal of the Movement Disorder Society, 26*(Suppl. 3), S42−S80.

Setthawatcharawanich, S., Limapichat, K., Sathirapanya, P., & Phabphal, K. (2011). Validation of the Thai SCOPA-sleep scale for assessment of sleep and sleepiness in patients with Parkinson's disease. *Journal of the Medical Association of Thailand = Chotmaihet Thangphaet, 94*(2), 179−184.

Shpirer, I., Miniovitz, A., Klein, C., Goldstein, R., Prokhorov, T., Theitler, J., et al. (2006). Excessive daytime sleepiness in patients with Parkinson's disease: A polysomnography study. *Movement Disorders: Official Journal of the Movement Disorder Society, 21*(9), 1432−1438.

Simuni, T., Caspell-Garcia, C., Coffey, C., Chahine, L. M., Lasch, S., Oertel, W. H., et al. (2015). Correlates of excessive daytime sleepiness in de novo Parkinson's disease: A case control study. *Movement Disorders: Official Journal of the Movement Disorder Society, 30*(10), 1371−1381.

Sobreira-Neto, M. A., Pena-Pereira, M. A., Sobreira, E. S. T., Chagas, M. H. N., Fernandes, R. M. F., Tumas, V., et al. (2017). High frequency of sleep disorders in

Parkinson's disease and its relationship with quality of life. *European Neurology, 78*(5−6), 330−337.

Stavitsky, K., & Cronin-Golomb, A. (2011). Sleep quality in Parkinson disease: An examination of clinical variables. *Cognitive and Behavioral Neurology: Official Journal of the Society for Behavioral and Cognitive Neurology, 24*(2), 43−49.

Stavitsky, K., Saurman, J. L., McNamara, P., & Cronin-Golomb, A. (2010). Sleep in Parkinson's disease: A comparison of actigraphy and subjective measures. *Parkinsonism & Related Disorders, 16*(4), 280−283.

Stefansdottir, S., Gjerstad, M. D., Tysnes, O. B., & Larsen, J. P. (2012). Subjective sleep problems in patients with early Parkinson's disease. *European Journal of Neurology: The Official Journal of the European Federation of Neurological Societies, 19*(12), 1575−1581.

Suzuki, K., Miyamoto, T., Miyamoto, M., Okuma, Y., Hattori, N., Kamei, S., et al. (2008). Excessive daytime sleepiness and sleep episodes in Japanese patients with Parkinson's disease. *Journal of the Neurological Sciences, 271*(1−2), 47−52.

Suzuki, K., Miyamoto, M., Miyamoto, T., Okuma, Y., Hattori, N., Kamei, S., et al. (2009). Correlation between depressive symptoms and nocturnal disturbances in Japanese patients with Parkinson's disease. *Parkinsonism & Related Disorders, 15*(1), 15−19.

Suzuki, K., Okuma, Y., Hattori, N., Kamei, S., Yoshii, F., Utsumi, H., et al. (2007). Characteristics of sleep disturbances in Japanese patients with Parkinson's disease. A study using Parkinson's disease sleep scale. *Movement Disorders: Official Journal of the Movement Disorder Society, 22*(9), 1245−1251.

Taus, C., Giuliani, G., Pucci, E., D'Amico, R., & Solari, A. (2003). Amantadine for fatigue in multiple sclerosis. *The Cochrane Database of Systematic Reviews*, (2), CD002818. doi(2), CD002818.

Thannickal, T. C., Lai, Y. Y., & Siegel, J. M. (2007). Hypocretin (orexin) cell loss in Parkinson's disease. *Brain: Journal of Neurology, 130*(Pt 6), 1586−1595.

Trotti, L. M., & Bliwise, D. L. (2010). No increased risk of obstructive sleep apnea in Parkinson's disease. *Movement Disorders: Official Journal of the Movement Disorder Society, 25*(13), 2246−2249.

Uc, E. Y., Rizzo, M., Anderson, S. W., Sparks, J. D., Rodnitzky, R. L., & Dawson, J. D. (2006). Driving with distraction in Parkinson disease. *Neurology, 67*(10), 1774−1780.

Valko, P. O., Waldvogel, D., Weller, M., Bassetti, C. L., Held, U., & Baumann, C. R. (2010). Fatigue and excessive daytime sleepiness in idiopathic Parkinson's disease differently correlate with motor symptoms, depression and dopaminergic treatment. *European Journal of Neurology: The Official Journal of the European Federation of Neurological Societies, 17*(12), 1428−1436.

Verbaan, D., Marinus, J., Visser, M., van Rooden, S. M., Stiggelbout, A. M., & van Hilten, J. J. (2007). Patient-reported autonomic symptoms in Parkinson disease. *Neurology, 69*(4), 333−341.

Verbaan, D., van Rooden, S. M., van Hilten, J. J., & Rijsman, R. M. (2010). Prevalence and clinical profile of restless legs syndrome in Parkinson's disease. *Movement Disorders: Official Journal of the Movement Disorder Society, 25*(13), 2142−2147.

Verbaan, D., van Rooden, S. M., Visser, M., Marinus, J., Emre, M., & van Hilten, J. J. (2009). Psychotic and compulsive symptoms in Parkinson's disease. *Movement Disorders: Official Journal of the Movement Disorder Society, 24*(5), 738−744.

Verbaan, D., van Rooden, S. M., Visser, M., Marinus, J., & van Hilten, J. J. (2008). Nighttime sleep problems and daytime sleepiness in Parkinson's disease. *Movement Disorders: Official Journal of the Movement Disorder Society, 23*(1), 35–41.

Viallet, F., Pitel, S., Lancrenon, S., & Blin, O. (2013). Evaluation of the safety and tolerability of rasagiline in the treatment of the early stages of Parkinson's disease. *Current Medical Research and Opinion, 29*(1), 23–31.

Videnovic, A., Klerman, E. B., Wang, W., Marconi, A., Kuhta, T., & Zee, P. C. (2017). Timed light therapy for sleep and daytime sleepiness associated with Parkinson disease: A randomized clinical trial. *JAMA Neurology, 74*(4), 411–418.

Videnovic, A., Noble, C., Reid, K. J., Peng, J., Turek, F. W., Marconi, A., et al. (2014). Circadian melatonin rhythm and excessive daytime sleepiness in Parkinson disease. *JAMA Neurology, 71*(4), 463–469.

Visser, M., van Rooden, S. M., Verbaan, D., Marinus, J., Stiggelbout, A. M., & van Hilten, J. J. (2008). A comprehensive model of health-related quality of life in Parkinson's disease. *Journal of Neurology, 255*(10), 1580–1587.

Wang, G., Wan, Y., Cheng, Q., Xiao, Q., Wang, Y., Zhang, J., et al. (2010). Malnutrition and associated factors in Chinese patients with Parkinson's disease: Results from a pilot investigation. *Parkinsonism & Related Disorders, 16*(2), 119–123.

Watts, R. L., Jankovic, J., Waters, C., Rajput, A., Boroojerdi, B., & Rao, J. (2007). Randomized, blind, controlled trial of transdermal rotigotine in early Parkinson disease. *Neurology, 68*(4), 272–276.

Weerkamp, N. J., Tissingh, G., Poels, P. J., Zuidema, S. U., Munneke, M., Koopmans, R. T., et al. (2013). Nonmotor symptoms in nursing home residents with Parkinson's disease: Prevalence and effect on quality of life. *Journal of the American Geriatrics Society, 61*(10), 1714–1721.

Weintraub, D., Mavandadi, S., Mamikonyan, E., Siderowf, A. D., Duda, J. E., Hurtig, H. I., et al. (2010). Atomoxetine for depression and other neuropsychiatric symptoms in Parkinson disease. *Neurology, 75*(5), 448–455.

Wienecke, M., Werth, E., Poryazova, R., Baumann-Vogel, H., Bassetti, C. L., Weller, M., et al. (2012). Progressive dopamine and hypocretin deficiencies in Parkinson's disease: Is there an impact on sleep and wakefulness? *Journal of Sleep Research, 21*(6), 710–717.

Yong, M. H., Fook-Chong, S., Pavanni, R., Lim, L. L., & Tan, E. K. (2011). Case control polysomnographic studies of sleep disorders in Parkinson's disease. *PLoS One, 6*(7), e22511.

Zhu, K., van Hilten, J. J., & Marinus, J. (2014). Predictors of dementia in Parkinson's disease; findings from a 5-year prospective study using the SCOPA-COG. *Parkinsonism & Related Disorders, 20*(9), 980–985.

Zhu, K., van Hilten, J. J., Putter, H., & Marinus, J. (2013). Risk factors for hallucinations in Parkinson's disease: Results from a large prospective cohort study. *Movement Disorders: Official Journal of the Movement Disorder Society, 28*(6), 755–762.

Brief reference on sleep staging

Sleep, as captured via polysomnography, is stageable based on certain characteristics derived from electroencephalogram (EEG), electrooculogram (EOG), electromyogram (EMG), heart rate data, and respiratory data. Broadly, sleep stages include rapid eye movement (REM) and non-REM (NREM). NREM is further divided into three stages: stage N1, stage N2, and stage N3.

A predictable progression of sleep stages over the night is seen in the majority of healthy, normal young adults. Further information on sleep stages and their progression over the night in normal young adults is shown in Table 13.1 (Ohayon, Carskadon, Guilleminault, & Vitiello, 2004). Sleep architecture is the general term used to refer to the characteristics of sleep as ascertained via polysomnography, in relation to sleep-onset latency, sleep time, and distribution of sleep stages. The polysomnographically defined sleep stages include stage N1 ("light" sleep), stage N2, stage N3 (slow wave sleep, "deep" sleep, or delta sleep), and REM sleep. In a normal healthy adult without sleep comorbidities or sleep deprivation, sleep usually starts with stage N1 and progresses over the night in cycles. A hypnogram is a visual depiction of the distribution of sleep stages over a given night, again as assessed on polysomnography. Sample hypnograms from one-night polysomnography from PD patients, and depicting some of these sleep architecture changes that can be seen, are shown in Fig. 13.1.

Predictable changes in sleep architecture occur with increasing age. Sleep latency increases, percent of sleep time spent in stage N1 and stage N2 increases, and percent of REM sleep diseases (Ohayon, Carskadon, Guilleminault, & Vitiello, 2004).

Changes in sleep architecture in Parkinson's disease

When interpreting data on sleep architecture changes in PD, it is important to consider the sample under investigation. Some studies have compared a "general" sample of PD to non-PD controls. On the other hand, other studies have compared PD patients with versus without "good" sleep, and definitions of the latter have varied across studies as well but are often based on subjective determination by the patient. With that in mind, there are contradictory data on whether PD patients have less REM sleep as compared with non-PD controls, with some studies finding

Disorders of Sleep and Wakefulness in Parkinson's Disease. https://doi.org/10.1016/B978-0-323-67374-7.00013-4

Table 13.1 Sleep stage definition and architecture in normal young adults.

	Other names	Progression over the night	Polysomnographic characteristics	Proportion of sleep	Comments
Stage N1	Stage 1	Usually the stage of sleep most people enter into during initial sleep	Slow rolling eye movements, mixed-frequency low-amplitude EEG in theta range (4–7 Hz) for at least half of a 30-s period	5%–10% of total sleep time	Lightest stage of sleep
Stage N2	Stage 2	Usually follows stage N1 and continues throughout the night off and on	4–7 Hz EEG with either sleep spindles or K-complexes. Spindles are brief bursts (<0.5 seconds) of increased EEG activity in the 11–16 Hz range that most often occur over the vertex. K-complexes are negative sharp waves followed by a positive component that last 0.5 seconds or more. They are usually most prominent over the frontal regions	45%–55%	Most of sleep is spent in stage N2
Stage N3	Stage 3, slow-wave sleep, delta sleep (encompasses what was previously labeled stage 4)	More likely to occur in first half of night	0.5–2 Hz EEG frequencies that are high amplitude (>75 μV) for 20% or more of a 30-second period	10%–20%	"Deep" sleep
REM sleep	Stage R	Occurs every 90–120 minutes; duration of REM episodes occurs during second half of night. Sleep-onset REM occurs with sleep deprivation and narcolepsy. Depression is associated with reduced REM latency	Low-voltage mixed-frequency on EEG with sawtooth waves. Sawtooth waves are brief bursts of 2–6 Hz waves with sharp contours. EMG shows atonia (loss of EMG activity) although intermittent phasic bursts of low-amplitude EMG activity are normal. EOG shows REMs: conjugate, sharply peaked eye movements	18%–23%	Stage during which vivid dreams are more likely to occur

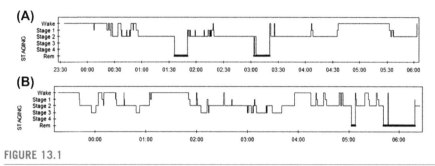

FIGURE 13.1

Hypnogram from a patient with Parkinson's disease (PD). (A) A prolonged sleep-onset latency and absence of stage 3 sleep is seen. (B) Apparent from this hypnogram is a delayed rapid eye movement (REM) latency.

this (Breen et al., 2014; Buskova et al., 2011; Shpirer et al., 2006; Yong, Fook-Chong, Pavanni, Lim, & Tan, 2011), but others not (Cochen De Cock et al., 2010; Diederich, Rufra, Pieri, Hipp, & Vaillant, 2013). Some studies have also found reduced sleep efficiency in PD compared with non-PD controls (Breen et al., 2014; Brunner et al., 2002; Happe et al., 2004), increased sleep latency (Breen et al., 2014), increased REM latency (Yong et al., 2011), and decreased total sleep time (Happe et al., 2004). On the other hand, none of these findings are consistent (Mantovani, Smith, Gordon, & O'Sullivan, 2018). Indeed, studies have also found both increases, decreases, and no difference in amount of stage 2 and stage 3 sleep in PD compared with non-PD controls (Mantovani et al., 2018). These differences may in part be accounted for by differences in environment of sleep assessment, by effects of PD disease stage (Mantovani et al., 2018), as well as by the effect of dopaminergic (and other) medications (Mantovani et al., 2018; Wailke, Herzog, Witt, Deuschl, & Volkmann, 2011). Further complicating interpretation of sleep architecture changes in PD is the effect of medications (Table 13.2). The majority of data on effects of medications on sleep architecture was obtained on healthy young adult samples. To what degree the disease process in PD changes the effects of these medications on sleep architecture is not known but must be considered in interpretation of these data. This is particularly true for dopaminergic medications. In the non-PD population, dopamine generally enhances wakefulness/inhibits sleep. However, the effects of dopamine on sleep may be dose dependent. For example, animal data indicate that low doses of dopaminergic medications facilitate sleep through action at presynaptic D2 receptors, whereas higher doses inhibit sleep through action at postsynaptic D1 and possibly also D2 receptors (Laloux et al., 2008; Monti, Hawkins, Jantos, D'Angelo, & Fernandez, 1988; Monti, Jantos, & Fernandez, 1989). In PD, divergent effects of dopamine on sleep and wakefulness in relation to dose and the underlying disease are seen (Bliwise et al., 2012). Therefore, generalized statements regarding effects of dopamine on sleep and wakefulness in PD simply cannot be made.

Table 13.2 Effect of medications on sleep architecture (with emphasis on meds used in PD[a]).

	Effect on NREM	Effect on REM
Dopaminergic agents		
Benzodiazepines	Increase stage N2 sleep, increase fast activity	
Nonbenzodiazepine receptor agonists	Reduce stage N1 sleep, increase stage N2 sleep	May reduce REM sleep
Alcohol		Delay and/or decrease REM sleep
MAO inhibitors		Delay and/or decrease REM sleep
Selective serotonin reuptake inhibitors	Increase stage N1 sleep	Delay and/or decrease REM sleep
Serotonin antagonist and reuptake inhibitor (trazodone)	Increase stage N3 (slow-wave) sleep	
Serotonin norepinephrine reuptake inhibitors		Delay and/or decrease REM sleep
Tricyclic antidepressants	Increase stage N3 (slow-wave) sleep	Decrease REM sleep
Sedative hypnotics		Delay and/or decrease REM sleep
Anticholinergics		Delay and/or decrease REM sleep
Opioids	Decrease stage N3 (slow-wave) sleep	Decrease REM sleep
Melatonin and melatonin receptor agonists	Reduce stage N1 sleep	Decrease REM sleep
Lithium	Increases stage N3 (slow-wave) sleep	Decrease REM sleep
Atypical antipsychotics	Increase stage N3 (slow-wave) sleep	
Beta-blockers		Decrease REM sleep
Anticonvulsants	Carbamazepine increases stage N1 and stage N2 sleep. Gabapentin increases stage N3 (slow wave) sleep	Carbamazepine decreases REM sleep Phenobarbital decreases REM sleep
Alpha 2 delta ligands	Increase stage N3 (slow-wave) sleep	

NREM, *non-REM*; PD, *Parkinson's disease*; REM, *rapid eye movement*.
[a] *The majority of data on effects of medications on sleep architecture is in healthy young adult samples. To what degree the disease process in PD changes the effects of these medications on sleep architecture is not known but must be considered in interpretation of these data.*

Subjective sleep and objective sleep are not well correlated in PD. This also is likely accounted for by various factors, including the artificial environment of the sleep lab and research environment in general (as compared with the typical environment the patient sleeps in), the somewhat artificial division of sleep into sleep stages on polysomnography, and the lack of accounting for in night-to-night variability often seen in one-night in-lab polysomnography studies (which account for the majority of studies on objective sleep measurement in PD).

References

Bliwise, D. L., Trotti, L. M., Wilson, A. G., Greer, S. A., Wood-Siverio, C., Juncos, J. J., et al. (2012). Daytime alertness in Parkinson's disease: Potentially dose-dependent, divergent effects by drug class. *Movement Disorders: Official Journal of the Movement Disorder Society, 27*(9), 1118–1124.

Breen, D. P., Vuono, R., Nawarathna, U., Fisher, K., Shneerson, J. M., Reddy, A. B., et al. (2014). Sleep and circadian rhythm regulation in early Parkinson disease. *JAMA Neurology, 71*(5), 589–595.

Brunner, H., Wetter, T. C., Hogl, B., Yassouridis, A., Trenkwalder, C., & Friess, E. (2002). Microstructure of the non-rapid eye movement sleep electroencephalogram in patients with newly diagnosed Parkinson's disease: Effects of dopaminergic treatment. *Movement Disorders: Official Journal of the Movement Disorder Society, 17*(5), 928–933.

Buskova, J., Klempir, J., Majerova, V., Picmausova, J., Sonka, K., Jech, R., et al. (2011). Sleep disturbances in untreated Parkinson's disease. *Journal of Neurology, 258*(12), 2254–2259.

Cochen De Cock, V., Abouda, M., Leu, S., Oudiette, D., Roze, E., Vidailhet, M., et al. (2010). Is obstructive sleep apnea a problem in Parkinson's disease? *Sleep Medicine, 11*(3), 247–252.

Diederich, N. J., Rufra, O., Pieri, V., Hipp, G., & Vaillant, M. (2013). Lack of polysomnographic Non-REM sleep changes in early Parkinson's disease. *Movement Disorders: Official Journal of the Movement Disorder Society, 28*(10), 1443–1446.

Happe, S., Anderer, P., Pirker, W., Klosch, G., Gruber, G., Saletu, B., et al. (2004). Sleep microstructure and neurodegeneration as measured by [123I]beta-CIT SPECT in treated patients with Parkinson's disease. *Journal of Neurology, 251*(12), 1465–1471.

Laloux, C., Derambure, P., Houdayer, E., Jacquesson, J. M., Bordet, R., Destee, A., et al. (2008). Effect of dopaminergic substances on sleep/wakefulness in saline- and MPTP-treated mice. *Journal of Sleep Research, 17*(1), 101–110.

Mantovani, S., Smith, S. S., Gordon, R., & O'Sullivan, J. D. (2018). An overview of sleep and circadian dysfunction in Parkinson's disease. *Journal of Sleep Research, 27*(3), e12673.

Monti, J. M., Hawkins, M., Jantos, H., D'Angelo, L., & Fernandez, M. (1988). Biphasic effects of dopamine D-2 receptor agonists on sleep and wakefulness in the rat. *Psychopharmacology, 95*(3), 395–400.

Monti, J. M., Jantos, H., & Fernandez, M. (1989). Effects of the selective dopamine D-2 receptor agonist, quinpirole on sleep and wakefulness in the rat. *European Journal of Pharmacology, 169*(1), 61–66.

Ohayon, M. M., Carskadon, M. A., Guilleminault, C., & Vitiello, M. V. (2004). Meta-analysis of quantitative sleep parameters from childhood to old age in healthy individuals: Developing normative sleep values across the human lifespan. *Sleep, 27*(7), 1255–1273.

Shpirer, I., Miniovitz, A., Klein, C., Goldstein, R., Prokhorov, T., Theitler, J., et al. (2006). Excessive daytime sleepiness in patients with Parkinson's disease: A polysomnography study. *Movement Disorders: Official Journal of the Movement Disorder Society, 21*(9), 1432–1438.

Wailke, S., Herzog, J., Witt, K., Deuschl, G., & Volkmann, J. (2011). Effect of controlled-release levodopa on the microstructure of sleep in Parkinson's disease. *European Journal of Neurology: The Official Journal of the European Federation of Neurological Societies, 18*(4), 590–596.

Yong, M. H., Fook-Chong, S., Pavanni, R., Lim, L. L., & Tan, E. K. (2011). Case control polysomnographic studies of sleep disorders in Parkinson's disease. *PLoS One, 6*(7), e22511.

Index

Printed and bound by CPI Group (UK) Ltd, Croydon, CR0 4YY

03/10/2024

01040349-0008